QUALITY ASSURANCE IN HOSPITAL PHARMACY

Strategies and Techniques

Marlene Lamnin, B.Sc.
Director of Quality Assurance
HPI Hospital Pharmacies

Contributing Author
Gary L. Snodgrass, Pharm.D., M.Ed.
Director of Clinical Services
HPI Hospital Pharmacies

AN ASPEN PUBLICATION®
Aspen Systems Corporation
Rockville, Maryland
London
1983

The author(s) has (have) endeavored to provide drug administration guidelines that are in agreement with current literature. It is suggested that appropriate information sources be consulted when dealing with new and unfamiliar drugs. It remains the responsibility of every practitioner to evaluate the appropriateness of a particular opinion in the context of the actual clinical situation with due consideration to any new developments in the field of drug administration.

Library of Congress Cataloging in Publication Data

Lamnin, Marlene.
Quality assurance in hospital pharmacy.

Bibliography.
Includes index.
1. Hospital pharmacies—Quality control.
2. Quality assurance. I. Snodgrass, Gary N.
II. Title. [DNLM: 1. Pharmacy service, hospital—Standards. 2. Quality assurance, health care.
WX179 L232q]
RA975.5.P5L35 1983 362.1'782'0685 82-18167
ISBN: 0-89443-925-1

Publisher: John Marozsan
Editorial Director: Michael Brown
Managing Editor: Margot Raphael
Editorial Services: Eileen Higgins
Printing and Manufacturing: Debbie Collins

Illustrator: Terri Asher

Library of Congress Catalog Card Number: 82-18167
ISBN: 0-89443-925-1

Printed in the United States of America

1 2 3 4 5

To my family, friends, and coworkers,
whose belief in me gives me strength.

Table of Contents

Preface

Quality Assurance Applied to Hospital Pharmacy has been written from the perspective of a hospital pharmacist. The principles of quality assurance that are presented, however, apply to any institutional health care service. Professionals in all health disciplines should be able to apply the concepts of quality assurance to the functions of any hospital department. Quality assurance must be an integral component of every patient care service. Throughout the text, quality assurance is referred to as a management tool. The material that follows is meant to be of practical value to the reader and a guide to the use of this tool.

Marlene Lamnin, B.Sc.
December 1982

Preface

Acknowledgments

Good fortune is often attributed to being in the right place at the right time. There is no doubt that the opportunity to write this book can be placed in that category. By assuming the directorship of the QA program for HPI Hospital Pharmacies, Inc., I was able to observe the nationwide awakening to the need for quality assurance and the development of innovative techniques to meet that need. It was my hope that by writing this book I would be able to share my experience and observations with those who are charged with the responsibility of providing QA activities in hospitals.

Before I could even accept the assignment from Aspen Systems Corporation to write this text, I needed to obtain approval from two sources: my family and my employer. My husband, Joseph, and my daughter, Sara, agreed to allow me the time to research and write the chapters and provided encouragement and assistance along the way. My employer, HPI Hospital Pharmacies, Inc., and particularly my boss, A. Clifford Better, generously offered professional support and permitted the inclusion of parts of HPI's comprehensive QA program.

It became obvious while designing the content outline that a chapter on the subject of clinical pharmacy services was necessary. My colleague, Dr. Gary Snodgrass, Director of Clinical Services for HPI, consented to write this chapter, despite his many other commitments. Not to be forgotten are the patience and attention to detail of our secretary, Alice Riley.

Other experts, both within HPI and in related health care fields, reviewed specific chapters and added their knowledge. It has been said that if you need a task accomplished, assign it to a busy person. In the case of these reviewers, this maxim was certainly true. For finding the time to share their expertise, I wish to express my special thanks to Pauline Canter, Director of Nursing Services; Robert Kass, Director of Purchasing for HPI; and Richard Yisha, President of Euclid Medical Systems and Euclid Pharmaceuticals, Inc. By providing me with their viewpoints, these individuals broadened the scope and depth of the content they reviewed.

A work of this type does not develop in a vacuum. Each practitioner I have met, each article I have read, and each seminar I have attended have been beneficial. In addition, I have had the unique opportunity, while serving as HPI's Director of Quality Assurance, to travel to most of our contract pharmacy and materiel management departments. I have found it very gratifying to observe the various creative methods used to solve common problems. Many of the examples cited throughout the book come from actual experiences in HPI facilities.

I am indebted to my sister, Zelda Provenzano, who is a teacher and professional editor, for painstakingly editing each chapter before the final manuscript was typed to improve the grammar and ensure continuity. Without her help, my modifiers would remain misplaced and my infinitives permanently split. The illustrations were created by Terri Asher, an artist who lives in Los Angeles and is skilled in cartooning and graphics.

One last set of acknowledgments is in order: to Terry Trudeau, editor of *Topics in Hospital Pharmacy Management*, Mike Brown and Sandy Cannon of Aspen Systems Corporation, my thanks for inviting me to prepare the text, for convincing Aspen Systems Corporation of the need for a book on this subject, and for assisting me with the technical details of manuscript preparation.

To everyone who provided assistance, encouragement, and support during the writing process, I extend my humble and heartfelt gratitude.

Part I

Overview of Quality Assurance

Chapter 1

Why Quality Assurance?

1

Patients receiving medical care in hospitals, whether by choice or by accident, place their trust in the professionals responsible for providing treatment. Quality Assurance is one of the mechanisms available to ensure that a consistently high level of health care is provided continuously. Quality Assurance (QA) is a method used to identify problems and to document that the problems are corrected.

The literature is replete with shocking accounts of harm done to patients in hospitals having few or no monitoring controls. A few examples are given below:

- In 1976, seven pediatric patients developed septicemia after receiving intravenous solutions containing potassium chloride, which had been added by the hospital pharmacist. The causative organism, *Enterobacter aerogenes*, identified by culture, was present in five of the pharmacy employees. To further complicate the situation, the admixtures were left at room temperature after compounding and some were not administered for several days after preparation.[1]
- Twenty-two patients developed fungemia caused by *Candida parapsilosis* in parenteral nutrition solutions prepared in the pharmacy department. The vacuum system, used to withdraw fluids and facilitate addition of medications, was found to be the source of the organism.[2] Incorrect use of the vacuum allowed a back flow of the intravenous solution into the pump tubing, where the *Candida* had colonized.
- The "Medication Error Reports" column in *Hospital Pharmacy* prints drug errors every month, along with a discussion of the cause and possible prevention methods. Error no. 48 described a situation in which 0.625-mg conjugated estrogens (Premarin) tablets were prescribed.[3] The technician reading the order apparently thought that the physician ordered 6.25 mg and decided to give an equivalent dose by dispensing five 1.25-mg tablets at one

> time in the patient's unit dose bin. The error went undetected by the pharmacist. When the nurse questioned the use of five tablets, the technician assured the nurse that the five-tablet dosage was correct. Again, there was no intervention by the pharmacist. Three days after the dose was administered, the patient, who had a history of gynecological problems, developed vaginal bleeding.

These examples point out the need for an active control system in every area of pharmacy performance. As early as 1962, when the American Society of Hospital Pharmacists (ASHP) published its "Statement on the Abilities Required of Hospital Pharmacists," quality control in hospital pharmacy was recognized as an essential component of institutional practice.[4] The statement included, among other abilities, the following, which relate to controls: quality assurance of drugs purchased and dispensed, internal controls for drug dispensing, and control of drugs located in the hospital, outside the pharmacy.

Referring to this ASHP statement, Lamy added other areas for consideration, such as prepackaging medications and cleaning and maintaining equipment.[5] The basic concepts of quality assurance for the hospital pharmacist were defined and explained by Stolar in the *American Journal of Hospital Pharmacy*.[6-8] Stolar's work has provided a strong foundation for building a comprehensive QA program.

Other recent events have focused the spotlight on QA activities in hospital pharmacies. The first, in 1971, was the incidence of contaminated intravenous fluids, which resulted in a national recall of the solutions.[9] The National Coordinating Committee on Large Volume Parenterals (NCCLVP) was formed to review problems in intravenous therapy and to recommend corrective actions. The statements issued by this multidisciplinary group have provided guidelines for every phase of manufacturing, dispensing, and administration of intravenous solutions. The current Good Manufacturing Practices Act was promulgated in 1978 to prevent the recurrence of this dangerous situation.[10]

The second circumstance to have an impact on recognition of the value of quality assurance was the implementation of a requirement for a QA program as a prerequisite for accreditation by the Joint Commission on Accreditation of Hospitals (JCAH).[11] Published in the 1980 *Accreditation Manual for Hospitals*, the standard became effective on January 1, 1981. It states:

> There shall be evidence of a well defined, organized program designed to enhance patient care through the ongoing, objective assessment of important aspects of patient care and the correction of identified problems. . . . the effectiveness of a hospital's QA program shall be emphasized in determining a hospital's accreditation status.

It seems that *quality assurance* has become the latest "buzz word" in health care. The majority of seminars, newsletters, and journals list at least one QA topic. However, unlike many valid concepts whose popularity waxes and wanes, QA techniques have been used for centuries.

One of the earliest recorded examples of physician accountability took place during the reign of King Hammurabi, who ruled Babylon in 1800 B.C. If a surgeon was responsible for a patient's death or blindness, the law required that the surgeon forfeit a hand.[12]

Until A.D. 500 to 700, the Visigoths in France and Spain required physicians to post a security fee *before* treatment was initiated. If treatment was successful, the deposit was returned and the physician's fee was paid. If the patient died, the physician forfeited his investment and was forced to spend a mourning period with the family of the deceased.[13] Even Florence Nightingale played a role in collecting data: she is credited with devising the first uniform reporting mechanism for hospital statistics.[14]

In more modern times, groups of professionals became involved with the quality of care being provided. The number of ingredients in the alphabet soup has increased over the years: JCAH, Professional Standards Review Organization (PSRO), ASHP, and NCCLVP. Each has added another dimension to the complex activities known collectively as quality assurance.

This mini-tour through the history of quality assurance brings us to the present and to the rebirth of interest in the subject. In an age when health care costs, along with every other facet of daily life, are escalating, quality assurance can and must help hospitals run more effectively and efficiently. The total cost for health care in the United States in 1979 was $212.1 billion, which represents about nine percent of the gross national product. The Health Care Financing Administration (HCFA) estimated that hospital costs for the same year totaled $85.3 billion and that drugs cost the consumers $17 billion.[15] More effective controls in the pharmacies of the nation's hospitals can produce a dramatic impact on health care expenditures.

Other chapters in this book will explain the principles of quality assurance, its components and its benefits. It is hoped that the reader will find not only the tools but also the motivation to "build a better QA plan."

NOTES

1. A.T. Davis et al., "Primary Bacteremia—Illinois," *Morbidity and Mortality Weekly Report* 24 (April 6, 1976): 110-115.

2. J.F. Plouffe et al., "Nosocomial Outbreak of *Candida parapsilosis* Fungemia Related to Intravenous Infusions," *Archives of Internal Medicine* 137 (1977): 1686-1689.

3. Michael R. Cohen, "Medication Error Report #48," *Hospital Pharmacy* 11, no. 4 (1976): 146.

4. "Statement on the Abilities Required of Hospital Pharmacists," *American Journal of Hospital Pharmacy* 19 (1962): 493-496.

5. P.P. Lamy, "How Good Is Quality Control in Hospital Pharmacy Practice?" *Hospital Pharmacy* 9 (1974): 134.

6. Michael H. Stolar, "Quality Assurance for Hospital Pharmacy, Part I: Basic Concepts," *American Journal of Hospital Pharmacy* 32 (1975): 276-280.

7. Michael H. Stolar, "Conceptual Framework for Drug Usage Review, Medical Audit and Other Patient Care Review Procedures," *American Journal of Hospital Pharmacy* 34 (1977): 139-145.

8. American Society of Hospital Pharmacists, *Model Quality Assurance Program for Hospital Pharmacies* (Washington, D.C.: American Society of Hospital Pharmacists, 1978).

9. W.M. Heller, "On Maturing," *American Journal of Hospital Pharmacy* 29 (1972): 550.

10. "Current Good Manufacturing Practices," *Federal Register*, September 28, 1978.

11. *Accreditation Manual for Hospitals* (Chicago: Joint Commission on Accreditation of Hospitals, 1980) Appendix B, pp. 151-154.

12. Paul N. Batalden, *Quality Assurance in Ambulatory Care* (Rockville, Md.: Aspen Systems Corp., 1980), pp. 1-4.

13. Ibid.

14. Ibid.

15. Richard Surface, ed., *The White Sheet* (Columbus, Ohio: Philips Roxane, February 1981), no. 2.

Chapter 2

Sources of Standards, Criteria, and Data

2

One approach to development of a QA program in a hospital pharmacy is to observe the external and internal controls, guidelines, regulations, and standards of practice that guide the operation of the department. Measuring how the department complies with these standards is the beginning of quality assessment.

EXTERNAL STANDARDS

By looking first at those governmental and professional organizations that mandate pharmacy regulations and guidelines, a network of existing standards can be observed. The Drug Enforcement Agency (DEA) regulations have established methods for purchasing, controlling, dispensing, and destroying controlled substances.[1] Record-keeping requirements are also specified, such as the need for a biannual inventory of controlled substances. These can form the basis for measurable QA standards for the activities relating to controlled drugs. Further refinements can be made after reviewing state and local regulations and hospital policies pertaining to these drugs.

The influence of the Food and Drug Administration (FDA) must not be overlooked.[2] The regulations established by this agency affect the quality of the drugs and devices provided to the patient. Investigational drugs, recalls, packaging and labeling requirements, and patient package inserts are but a few of the areas over which the FDA has jurisdiction.

Continuing on a federal level, the Occupational Safety and Health Administration (OSHA) has promulgated building codes and safety guidelines for hospitals to protect both the patient and the employees.[3] These regulations also affect the physical plant and safety practices of the pharmacy.

Public Law 92-603, the 1972 amendments to the Social Security Law, established the requirement for institutional review of health care services, in the form of Professional Standards Review Organizations (PSRO).[4] Much of the assessment activity in health care in the 1970s was motivated by the operation of regional PSROs.

Although the main emphasis of the PSRO is peer review of the physician's performance, the regulations do provide for review of services by health care practitioners other than physicians, using the same methodology for audits. Thus, activities of ancillary departments such as pharmacy must also be reviewed.[5]

The PSRO must ask the following questions pertaining to services being provided by a hospital:[6]

- Were the services and items provided to the patient medically necessary?
- Does the quality of the services meet professionally recognized standards of health care?
- Could the services and items be provided on an outpatient basis or in another institution at lower cost?

Medicare reviews of hospital care ensure that length of stay and treatments prescribed are appropriate for the patients' diagnoses. Pharmacy is involved in these reviews from a reimbursement point of view. Medications and services must meet the Medicare guidelines or face a challenge that the hospital must defend. In addition, those hospitals not having a Joint Commission on Accreditation of Hospitals (JCAH) inspection receive an audit visit from a Medicare inspector. Changes in federal financing programs have defunded PSROs and will reduce the frequency of Medicare QA inspection visits. It becomes even more important to conduct our own QA assessments, since these cutbacks reduce monitoring by external agencies.

State and local laws also determine how pharmacy is practiced. As state laws begin to recognize hospital pharmacy as a distinct entity, more specific references on such subjects as the role of students, interns, and technicians in various functions can be expected. Educational requirements for relicensure are established by state boards of pharmacy. Since laws are not uniform, each pharmacist will have to be aware of the requirements of his or her respective board of pharmacy.

The state of the art becomes the standard of practice. Before advances in communication and transportation brought the world to our doorsteps, community standards were used to evaluate peer performance. Now, however, national and even international developments shape the delivery of health care in the local environment. Organizations such as the American Society of Hospital Pharmacists (ASHP), the National Coordinating Committee on Large Volume Parenterals (NCCLVP), the American Pharmaceutical Association (APhA), and many more establish guidelines that are adapted as the conventional levels of practice throughout the United States.

No discussion of standards would be complete without mentioning the JCAH. Originally, statements published by this group were "minimum standards of practice" for medicine, nursing, and all other areas of institutional health care. The JCAH standards have become the accepted norms, despite the fact that accreditation by this commission is voluntary.

CORPORATE STANDARDS

Moving inward, away from external sources of standards, we reach a middle ground that not all hospital pharmacies encounter. It encompasses those requirements established by corporate management groups such as American Medical International (AMI), Hospital Corporation of America (HCA), and HPI Hospital Pharmacies, Inc.[7] Each has standards of operational performance and quality assurance by which management's effectiveness is measured. As in the external standards, these should also be reviewed for compliance in daily activities.

INTERNAL STANDARDS

Rules established internally are derived from such sources as the hospital by-laws; credentials for medical staff and other professionals; and hospital, department, and personnel policies and procedures. These rules detail the specific methods for day-to-day operations in each unit of the institution.

Constructing a QA program for the pharmacy (or any other department) is not unlike building any structure. A strong foundation is provided by the external laws and regulations. The framework is shaped by state-of-the-art guidelines. State and local regulations determine the placement of fixtures and utilities. Interaction with other professionals and departments is carried out via the doors and windows (i.e., the hospital bylaws, policies, and procedures). Enclosing and protecting the facility is the roof, the QA committee, which oversees all functions, ensures quality of care, and protects those within from liability risks.

To build this structure you need architectural blueprints (i.e., the QA plan). The tools are at hand: professional education and experience. Other resources are close by in the form of various community professionals and organizations. The literature abounds with accounts of methods others have employed to accomplish this objective.

Once the QA structure is operational, it will prove to be a useful feature of the facility. The effort expended in construction will be part of the educational experience. Benefits are many and will be discussed in a later chapter.

SOURCES OF DATA FOR AUDITS

Because quality assurance in hospitals is to have a "problem focus," information sources in the institution must be reviewed in order to discover the existing problems. Kaplan and Hopkins advise that data from these sources should be organized to identify problems and to assist in prioritizing them. The authors suggest that the hospital's QA program be designed to synthesize data from each QA activity with information from other internal and external data sources. Those problems having the most impact on patient care should be addressed and resolved first.[8] The subject of problem identification will be developed more fully in Chapter 3.

The most obvious source of information is the patient's own record—the chart. Medical records professionals can provide assistance in data collection from patients' charts. Audits provide a useful purpose for collecting all the volumes of documentation required by law and fostered by concerns for liability risks. Confidentiality must be maintained in using this information. Skillicorn has identified several other sources of information in addition to the medical record chart,[9] and still other sources have been delineated by Affeldt.[10] These sources are summarized in Exhibit 2-1.

Once research has begun, information will be found everywhere. Another benefit of this exercise is that valuable record-keeping activities can be identified and useless ones can be eliminated. Duplication of effort can also be detected in the process. One of the benefits of developing a QA plan is the streamlining of record-keeping and reporting functions. These will be highlighted in the other sections of this book.

ROLE OF THE DRUG UTILIZATION REVIEW IN THE QA PROGRAM

Until the advent of the new JCAH standard for a hospital-wide, problem-focused QA program, the mainstay of pharmacy assessment was the Drug Utilization Review (DUR). Just as clinical pharmacy services have taken us away from strictly distributive functions, the multidisciplinary emphasis on quality assurance has also opened new vistas for review.

How to conduct drug utilization reviews has been discussed in great detail in the literature. Guidelines for specific activities related to DURs are outlined in Chapter 15. The value of this audit mechanism must not be underestimated.

An often-quoted study was conducted in 1972 by Roberts and Visconti, who reviewed 1,000 cases in a 500-bed hospital.[11] Their findings revealed that 65 percent of patients receiving antibiotics either required no therapy or were receiv-

Exhibit 2-1 Data Sources for QA Problem Identification

Patients' medical record	Diagnostic reports (lab, radiology)
Morbidity/Mortality records	Financial records
Hospital committee reports	• liability claims
Prescription review	• disallowed charges
PSRO and other regional data	• reimbursement challenges
Process studies	• third party payer data
Outcome studies	Utilization review findings
Drug utilization reviews	Staff and patient interviews
Log books (surgery, E.R.)	Computer printouts
Direct observation of patient care	Accreditation survey reports
Critique reports, e.g., CPR, fire, disaster drill	Personnel records (turnover, exit interviews, absenteeism)
Nursing care plans	Management reports
Incident reports (safety, clinical)	Clinical data, e.g., lab test results

Sources: Stanley A. Skillicorn, *Quality and Accountability*. San Francisco: Editorial Consultants, Inc., 1980, pp. 20-21. Reprinted with permission.

John E. Affeldt, "The New QA Standard of the Joint Commission on Accreditation of Hospitals." *The Western Journal of Medicine*, February 1980, pp. 166-170. Reprinted with permission.

ing an inappropriate dose. Since 1972, prescribing habits have greatly improved. However, antibiotics still represent 20 to 50 percent of a pharmacy's total drug budget.[12] It has also been estimated that 5 percent of hospitalized patients who are given an antibiotic will experience an adverse reaction to the drug.[13] Therefore, the appropriate use of these medications affects patient safety and economics.

Various sources are available for selecting audit topics. If the pharmacy receives a computer printout showing utilization figures for specific drug entities, trends in prescribing can be identified. By consulting with the infection control officer, the pharmacist can correlate prescribing data with patterns of infections seen in the hospital.

Specific drug classes, especially in the antibiotic area, lend themselves to audit. Drugs with toxic potential, such as aminoglycosides, and costly agents, such as cephalosporins, are natural subjects for review. Pharmacists are becoming very adept at demonstrating via drug utilization reviews that a more specific drug can be prescribed, thus effecting savings and measurable cost benefits. Multiple antibiotic therapy is also a subject worthy of review.

Other categories of drugs are excellent subjects of study because of the dosing guidelines or critical nature of their pharmacologic effects. Reviews of drugs such as digoxin, theophylline, heparin, warfarin, and lidocaine have measurable therapeutic parameters, which produce meaningful results. Support by the clinical laboratory in the hospital is vital if monitoring of the patient is to be timely and effective.

The JCAH guidelines for pharmacy specify one DUR per quarter.[14] The inspectors are also looking for an ongoing program to monitor the appropriateness of antibiotic therapy. In addition, reaudits should be conducted to assess the effectiveness of corrective action.

In summary, DURs are often the first exposure that pharmacists have to auditing activities. They provide an opportunity for interaction with other professionals, an opportunity for saving the hospital and the patient money, a mechanism for assessing effectiveness of prescribing and patient response, and one method of meeting the JCAH requirement for monitoring drug therapy.

NOTES

1. Public Law 91-513, *Controlled Substances Act*, October 27, 1970.

2. *Federal Food Drug and Cosmetic Act*, 1938.

3. Public Law 91-596, *Occupational Safety and Health Act of 1970*, 29USE 651 et seq.

4. Public Law 96-603, Review Responsibility and Authority of Professional Standards Review Organizations (PSROs), Department of Health Education and Welfare, Health Care Financing Administration, 1972.

5. Patricia C. Ostrow and Elizabeth Jones, "Peer Review for Non-physicians," *Hospitals* 53 (December 1, 1979): 66-69.

6. Carl T. DeMarch, *Pharmacy and the Law* (Rockville, Md.: Aspen Systems Corp. 1975), p. 85.

7. Kenneth N. Horowitz and Marlene Lamnin, "Design and Implementation of a Quality Assurance Program for Pharmaceutical Services," *American Journal of Hospital Pharmacy* 37 (January 1980): 82-84.

8. Karen O. Kaplan and Julie M. Hopkins, *The QA Guide—A Resource for Hospital Quality Assurance* (Chicago: Joint Commission on Accreditation of Hospitals, 1980), p. 47.

9. Stanley A. Skillicorn, *Quality and Accountability* (San Francisco: Editorial Consultants, Inc., 1980), pp. 20-21.

10. John E. Affeldt, "The New Quality Assurance Standard of the Joint Commission on Accreditation of Hospitals," *The Western Journal of Medicine*, February 1980, pp. 166-170.

11. A.W. Roberts and J.A. Visconti, "The Rational and Irrational Use of Systemic Antimicrobial Drugs," *American Journal of Hospital Pharmacy* 29 (1972): 1054-1060.

12. Ibid.

13. Ibid.

14. *Accreditation Manual for Hospitals* (Chicago: Joint Commission on Accreditation of Hospitals, 1980), pp. 137-145.

SUGGESTED READINGS

Brandon, Brenda B., et al. "Drug Usage Screening Criteria." *American Journal of Hospital Pharmacy* 34 (1977): 146-151.

DeMarco, Carl T. *Pharmacy and the Law*. Rockville, Md.: Aspen Systems Corporation, 1975.

Ellinoy, Brian J., et al. "Pharmacy Audit of Patient Health Records—Feasibility and Usefulness of a Drug Surveillance System." *American Journal of Hospital Pharmacy* 29 (1972): 749-754.

Hendricks, Jacalyn Newman. *Audit Criteria for Drug Utilization Review*. Washington, D.C.: American Society of Hospital Pharmacists, 1981.

Kunin, Calvin M., and Efron, Herman Y. "Guidelines for Peer Review." *Journal of the American Medical Association,* March 7—May 2, 1977.

Model Quality Assurance Program for Hospital Pharmacies. Washington, D.C.: American Society of Hospital Pharmacists, 1978 and 1980.

Palumbo, Francis B., et al. "Detecting Prescribing Problems Through Drug Usage Review: A Case Study." *American Journal of Hospital Pharmacy* 34 (1977): 152-154.

Pierpaoli, Paul G., et al. "Antibiotic Use Control—An Institutional Model," *Drug Intelligence and Clinical Pharmacy* 10 (1976): 258-267.

Skillicorn, Stanley A. *Quality and Accountability*. San Francisco: Editorial Consultants, Inc., 1980.

Stolar, Michael H. "Conceptual Framework for Drug Usage Review, Medical Audit and Other Patient Care Review Procedures." *American Journal of Hospital Pharmacy* 34 (1977): 139-145.

Towery, O.B., and Brands, Alvira, B., eds. U.S. Department of Health, Education and Welfare, Public Health Services, National Institute of Mental Health. *Psychotropic Drugs—Approaches to Psychopharmacologic Drug Use*. Washington, D.C.: U.S. Government Printing Office, publication no. 017-024-00926-1, 1979.

Tremblay, Jacques. "Creating an Appropriate Climate for Drug Use Review." *American Journal of Hospital Pharmacy* 38 (1981): 212-215.

Chapter 3

Methodology

3

Quality happens when everyone does everything exactly right every time.

—Dr. Stanley A. Skillicorn

A review of the literature on quality assurance reveals a specific language used to describe audit activities. In order to facilitate the reader's understanding of QA techniques used in health care, a brief explanation of this terminology is presented.

STRUCTURE, PROCESS, AND OUTCOME ASSESSMENTS

In order to conduct a QA assessment, one must first decide what will be measured. There are three different, but related, answers to this question. To state it another way, structures indicate the *where,* process denotes the *how,* and outcome represents the *what,* depending upon which service is being measured.

Structures are the physical and operational components of an organization. They include the physical facilities, equipment, personnel, staffing patterns, resources, and administrative organization. Structure assessment is object centered. *Process* components show how these structural elements are used to deliver service. Daily functions in the department are processes. The *outcome* is the "bottom line"—the final results of the care rendered, using the structures and processes at hand.[1,2]

Outcome assessment is the type most often used in health care. It asks the question: "Was the therapeutic goal reached?" Use of this method requires that the surveyor establish the endpoint *before* the analysis can take place. In health care, overall patterns of service are usually the objects of study, as contrasted to individual patient situations. Therefore, outcome analysis provides the majority of useful data in hospitals. Outcome criteria in health care predict the optimal achievable health status that the patient should attain.[3]

CONCURRENT, PROSPECTIVE, AND RETROSPECTIVE AUDITS

The analysis of a specific activity can be conducted while the activity is taking place. This is a *concurrent* audit. It may be difficult to conduct, in some cases, because the data needed may not be available or because the activity does not lend itself to this type of assessment. From the standpoint of affecting patient care in a positive manner, however, concurrent audits are usually very effective; results of a concurrent assessment can be used to suggest changes in a patient's therapy that will affect the outcome of the care given. Concurrent review has been compared with the practice of preventive medicine: it can stop negative events from happening.

Prospective assessments are conducted after the intent to provide the service has been stated but before the actual delivery of the service takes place. Structure and process assessments can be conducted prospectively. Since the event must be completed for an outcome review, prospective audits are not applicable. Reviews of physicians' orders can make a definite impact on patient safety and length of hospital stay when conducted prospectively for patient drug allergy potential, significant drug interactions, and clinical efficacy.

Retrospective audits are used most often in health care. Patients' records and other data sources are usually more readily available after care has been rendered. This methodology uses previously recorded information, which depends upon completeness and accuracy of the records being reviewed. Assessments of this type are based on review of the outcomes of therapy. Although the results of this method of review do not improve therapy for the patients included in the study, the technique is still valuable for identifying problems and suggesting improvements for the future.[4,5]

It has been suggested that when implementing an assessment program, such as drug utilization review, methods involving retrospective audits should be used. Retrospective reviews permit the auditor to revise the program as needed, during the learning process, without affecting patient outcomes. Also, because aggregate data are analyzed, patterns of information develop as a result of retrospective appraisals; concurrent and prospective systems usually involve individual cases.[6]

Each of these methods for assessment has its value. Although most drug audits are retrospective, the pharmacist should be aware that in some instances one of the other types of audit may provide more relevant results.

HOW TO FOCUS ON PROBLEMS, OR HOW TO CONTROL THE CONTENTS OF PANDORA'S BOX

The wording of the Joint Commission on Accreditation of Hospitals (JCAH) standard for quality assurance requires evidence of "the correction of problems."[7] Thus the health care professional has been given a direction and goal for QA endeavors. Identifying a problem, correcting it, ensuring that it has been corrected, and then assessing the value of the resulting improvement in patient care illustrate the essence of quality assurance.

The simplest method for problem identification is to list known or suspected problems and the areas that need improvement. Brainstorming with others in the department can bring still more problems to the surface. Then, the list is prioritized by eliminating those situations that cannot be corrected by the pharmacy department alone (e.g., larger space or new equipment).

Willie Sutton, a notorious bank robber, when asked why he robbed banks, replied, "That's where the money is." Sutton's law states, "Look for problems where they are most likely to be."[8] It is also beneficial to select those problems that have the potential for the largest patient benefit. Keeping this particular outcome in mind will lead to the satisfaction resulting from the correction of a real problem. It will be easier to obtain cooperation from others (on an audit or in another endeavor) if the benefits of the efforts are real, measurable, and positive.

The technique of identifying a problem and correcting the situation to prevent recurrence can be extended into other areas of management as well. For example, the "Smokey the Bear" management style channels efforts into crisis management rather than into prevention. A retrospective review of recent crises can provide insight into causes and into related preventative measures that can be implemented. The time saved in fighting fewer fires will enable the manager to develop plans for future activities and to provide a real impact on the effectiveness of the department's efforts. Moreover, problem identification techniques, once mastered, can be used in almost any other area of health care.

Skillicorn, who is recognized as one of the early proponents of quality assurance in medical care, has discussed the subject of problem identification very thoroughly in his book *Quality and Accountability*. It is his belief that problems in patient care occur for two main reasons:[9]

1. Less than 5 percent of the patient care errors take place because of a deficiency in knowledge by professionals.
2. The majority of errors are due to carelessness, poor performance, or apathetic attitude.

Quality should be defined as an attitude that encourages perfection and considers errors in patient care unacceptable. According to Skillicorn, the attitude that errors are inevitable is at the root of much of the poor performance in health care.[10] He believes that to improve the quality of health care we must bring about a change in this attitude. Therefore, the elimination of error alone is not sufficient. Caring for and about the patient is vital and must be demonstrated.[11] These points must be remembered when designing corrective actions to solve identified problems.

Often, the problems identified in health care are *systems* problems, involving many departments and professionals. Fortunately, the JCAH multidisciplinary requirement for QA activities encourages professionals to work together to set criteria and to take corrective action.[12]

The concept of "generic screens," developed in 1977 for the California Medical Association and California Hospital Association, is used in physician peer review.[13] The generic screen is defined by Sherman as a "patient condition or patient care event that might signal one or more problems in the health care system."[14] This concept reinforces both the systems and multidisciplinary approaches to problem correction. It is an approach that could also be applied to pharmacy-based problems.

Only those problems that can be corrected should be selected, and areas that are functioning well should be avoided. In other words, "If it ain't broke, don't fix it."

HOW TO DEVELOP AUDIT CRITERIA AND STANDARDS

In order to assess performance, ideal or acceptable ranges of performance must be established. *Criteria* are preestablished elements against which components of the quality of service may be measured. A *standard* expresses the range of deviation from the criteria that will be acceptable.[15]

Explicit criteria are required for an effective QA program. They must be written *before* the assessment is conducted and so that the results are reproducible, given the same set of data. *Implicit* criteria are unstructured and therefore require individual judgment on the part of the surveyor. As a result, implicit criteria are rarely reliable or reproducible.[16] Screening criteria are kept to a minimum (usually no more than six) on any particular audit. They represent a selected number of critical elements that, if absent from the data being reviewed, cause it to be "flagged" for further review. When a large body of information or many individual elements have to be reviewed, screening criteria facilitate selecting those that merit closer inspection. Screening criteria are often used to evaluate outcomes.[17] In-depth criteria may be many in number and cover various aspects of the service. These criteria lend themselves to the analysis of processes.[18] Sherman explains that criteria should represent a threshold for action, that is, when deviation from established standards is detected, corrective action is begun.[19] Therefore, in light of these fundamental principles, we can summarize by saying that QA standards must be:

- relevant
- measurable
- able to use readily retrievable data
- specific and complete
- able to produce results that are reliable and reproducible.

An example of how this process might work in the pharmacy is given below.

An outcome audit is designed to determine how reliably the pharmacy staff records drug allergies on patient profiles. One month's profiles will be examined in a retrospective review. Since this will require the examination of many pieces of information, a screening criterion is designed. The standard is written to show a measurable outcome, that is, "All pharmacy patient profiles will have drug allergy information recorded completely." Any profiles without allergy information will "fall out" and be subjected to further analysis. The results of the audit will lead to:

- decision about whether a problem exists
- analysis of causes
- design of corrective action
- possible in-service training for pharmacy and nursing personnel to ensure both receipt and recording of allergy data in the pharmacy
- reaudit to determine whether the problem is corrected.

A prospective audit could be accomplished, using a standard that specifies that "no medication will be dispensed until the patient's drug allergy information is screened in the pharmacy." This can affect and improve the care of those patients currently in the hospital. Since the result of compliance to this standard can be observed, the pharmacy staff may be more willing to follow the established procedure.

Criteria setting for a multidisciplinary review must be done by the entire group involved in the process. If all those participating do not "buy in" at the beginning, it may be difficult to achieve cooperation. Cretin was quoted in the *Quality Review Bulletin* as saying, "Unless feedback about poor medical practices results in improved practices, the whole audit procedure may be a waste of time."[20]

Now that the *what, how,* and *where* have been explained, the building of a QA program can begin. After the surveyor has the problem identified, the standards written, and the data collected and analyzed, the appropriate corrective actions can be selected.

NOTES

1. Robert L. Mikeal, "A Study Protocol for Evaluating the Quality of Pharmaceutical Services," *American Journal of Hospital Pharmacy* 31 (1974): 657-659.

2. Michael H. Stolar, "Conceptual Framework for Drug Usage Review, Medical Audit and Other Patient Care Review Procedures," *American Journal of Hospital Pharmacy* 34 (1977): 139-145.

3. Charles M. Jacobs and Susan Weagly, *Measuring Quality of Patient Care: Rationale for Outcome Audit* (Cambridge, Mass.: Ballinger Publishing Company, 1976), p. 38.

4. Stolar, "Conceptual Framework," pp. 140-141.

5. Stolar, "Quality Assurance for Hospital Pharmacy," *American Journal of Hospital Pharmacy* 32 (1975): 276-280.

6. O.B. Towery and A. Brands, eds., *Psychotropic Drugs–Approaches to Psychopharmacologic Drug Use* (Washington, D.C.: U.S. Government Printing Office, 1979), publication no. 017-024-00926-1, pp. 8-17.

7. *Accreditation Manual for Hospitals* (Chicago: Joint Commission on Accreditation of Hospitals, 1980) Appendix B, pp. 151-154.

8. Richard P. Hoffman, "General Suggestions for Auditing Antibiotic Usage," *Hospital Pharmacy* 15, no. 3 (1980): 143-147.

9. Stanley A. Skillicorn, *Quality and Accountability* (San Francisco: Editorial Consultants, Inc., 1980), pp. 20, 21, and 23.

10. Ibid., p. 23.

11. Ibid., pp. 25-26.

12. Ibid., pp. 31 and 38.

13. Ibid., pp. 51-61.

14. Samuel R. Sherman, "Generic Screening: A System Approach to Patient Care Audit Studies," *The Western Journal of Medicine,* September 1979, pp. 256-258.

15. Stolar, "Conceptual Framework," p. 140.

16. Ibid.

17. Ibid.

18. Ibid.

19. Samuel R. Sherman, "Redefining the Elements of Quality Assurance," Patient Care Assessment Council Meeting, Los Angeles, California, October 26, 1979.

20. Barbara Wendorf, ed., "Is Quality Assurance Really Worth It?" *Quality Review Bulletin* 7, no. 2 (1981): 26.

Chapter 4

How To Select and Implement Corrective Actions To Solve Problems

4

To get the maximum attention, it's hard to beat a good, big mistake.
—*Gazette*

In Gilbert and Sullivan's *The Mikado*, the Emperor of Japan designs a system of justice in which "the punishment fits the crime." In designing corrective actions for problems revealed by QA audits, the solution should fit the problem. Then a reaudit should be conducted to ensure that the problem is really solved. Monitoring of the *problem,* and not the solution, is essential.

The Joint Commission on Accreditation of Hospitals (JCAH) standard for quality assurance was written without specific guidelines for corrective action for a specific reason. It was the intent of the Commission to stimulate creative thinking in designing problem-solving activities.

Usually, the first impulse of the professional is to design an educational program, or in-service training, to correct a deficiency. The value of such programs should not be underestimated. It must be remembered, however, that this is only one solution. Studies have shown that deficiencies in health care services are attributed to poor performance 94 to 95 percent of the time; lack of knowledge is responsible for only 5 to 6 percent of the inadequate delivery of care.[1,2]

TYPES OF CORRECTIVE ACTIONS

In general, corrective actions can be classified in the same manner in which assessment techniques are grouped: structure, process, and outcome activities. Examples of each type are given below:

Structure activities:

- staffing changes
- development of new, or change in existing, policy or procedure
- design of new forms; revision of existing forms
- change in facilities, equipment, space
- change in hours of service
- new mechanisms for information gathering and communications

Process activities:

- educational programs
- development and implementation of a new service
- new methods of communication (e.g., on-line computer capability)
- disciplinary action by management (e.g., limiting privileges of medical staff)
- reward for good performance (incentives).

Outcome activities:

- educational activities with outcome goals
- rewards for good performance (goals achieved)
- disciplinary activity by management.

There are areas of overlap in each of these types; for example, communication devices are both structure and process. As the list demonstrates, there are varied avenues open to the manager. Development of appropriate corrective action is another facet of quality assurance that challenges creativity and stimulates cooperation among professionals in various disciplines. Here again the concept of quality assurance as a multidisciplinary activity is fostered. If all departments involved in the problem are part of designing the solution, a higher degree of acceptance of the alterations being implemented can be expected. Human nature resists change; those who are involved in planning for reforms can be effective in motivating others to accept new methods.

With the advances in health care technology, sometimes the cure is worse than the disease. In correcting a problem, we must strive to prevent the solution from becoming too complex to be workable. It is tempting to use this creative opportunity to design a detailed action plan that could unintentionally discourage those who attempt to follow it.

SELECTION OF APPROPRIATE CORRECTIVE ACTION

In order to design or select the most effective corrective action for a particular problem, three variables must be examined and identified:[3]

1. the location of the problem (e.g., one department, hospital-wide, one specific shift)
2. the participants (e.g., nurses, physicians, pharmacists, technicians)
3. the type of problem (e.g., lack of knowledge, attitude, communications)

Remembering that Skillicorn suggests that most health care problems are systems failures, a multidisciplinary approach to the solution must be found.[4] This can also be true within the pharmacy department. For example, a dispensing error problem should be solved by those professionals and technical people involved in daily dispensing activities.

Although a problem may have many causes, not every cause is correctable. If a shortage of qualified health care professionals is attributed to the rural location of the hospital, moving the hospital to an urban location is not a reasonable solution. However, other more achievable alternatives can be explored, such as finding professionals in the community who are not in active practice and providing them with refresher courses.

Once the three variables of location, participants, and type of problem have been established, an action plan can be written. This plan should:

- be specific and detailed, listing each step to be taken, and its deadline
- be measurable, with regard to desired results
- list accountable individuals
- specify when reassessment will be conducted
- indicate to whom and when the results will be reported.

The old saw, "It is the squeakiest wheel that gets the grease," can be a useful guideline when selecting those who will motivate changes in existing systems. By placing the chronic complainer on the planning committee, it is possible to rechannel the negative energy into constructive actions. Pride of authorship will encourage the former complainer to convince others of the value of the new plan. Control must be maintained, however, or the complainer can destroy the positive atmosphere needed for problem solving.

The channels of communication must be kept open in all directions, both while designing and while implementing corrective action. Adjustments made along the way show that the planners are really responsive to the needs of those involved. Feedback is provided on the progress of the improvements as a morale booster. Sharing the satisfaction achieved by the correction of a problem can facilitate similar activities in the future.

IMPLEMENTATION OF CORRECTIVE ACTION—A CASE STUDY

To illustrate the principles delineated thus far, a case study involving a real problem in pharmacy operations is presented and the choices made to remedy the situation are explained.

In a 100-bed rural, general, acute care hospital, an audit of drug charges for surgical patients was conducted. Pharmacy, nursing service, business office, and medical records personnel participated in the survey. The results were reported to the QA Committee and to the administrator.

The audit showed that of the 50 patients' charts and discharge bills reviewed, 60 percent of the patients had been undercharged for drugs used in the operating or recovery room. The average undercharge was $10 per patient. In addition, a review of floor stock costs for these two areas during the study period showed a total of $1,000 dispensed to the units but not charged to the patient.

The QA Committee appointed the director of pharmacy services and the Operating Room/Recovery Room (OR/RR) nursing supervisor to work together to detect causes and recommend solutions. They were to report back to the QA Committee at its next meeting in 30 days.

Through daily monitoring, these two individuals discovered the following facts affecting dispensing and administration of OR/RR drugs:

- Floor stock quantities were checked once a month by pharmacy, during the nursing unit inspections.
- Nurses, anesthetists, and anesthesiologists tended to "hoard" drugs to cover emergencies when they were on call or when the pharmacy was closed.
- There was a 24- to 48-hour delay between the time surgery was performed and the time pharmacy received charges for drugs administered.
- There was no centralized drug storage area in surgery, which fostered private stocks of supplies in each operating suite.
- Each surgeon, anesthetist, and anesthesiologist required individualized stocks, supplies, and drugs.

A problem-solving session was scheduled, with both pharmacists and surgical personnel attending. With the understanding that this would be a constructive meeting, everyone agreed to brainstorm possible solutions. Briefly, these were the steps decided upon by the group and referred to the QA Committee and other appropriate decision makers for approval:

- New stock lists were devised and quantities of drugs were assigned, based on past usage records. These lists were to be reviewed and revised no less than every six months. Each anesthetist, anesthesiologist, and nursing supervisor had input on each respective list.
- A centralized area in surgery was established for drug stock. A refrigerator was moved into the area. The site selected was accessible to each operating suite and serviced readily by pharmacy as well.
- A procedure was developed in which the supervisor in the operating room notified pharmacy at the close of the surgical day. Charges were brought to the pharmacy, along with a composite list of drugs needed for replacement. Charges were tallied against the list; drug replacements were prepared and delivered to surgery within one hour of receipt in the pharmacy. A physical count was conducted as replacements were delivered to the stock storage area. Discrepancies were noted and given to the operating room supervisor. Since it had only been a few hours since the drugs in question were used, the supervisor could easily track and charge for missing items. Any shortages still not reconciled after 24 hours were charged to surgery, at acquisition cost.
- The policy and procedure were approved by all concerned. In-service training for nursing, anesthesiology, and pharmacy staff members was conducted jointly, around the clock, for two days. Written copies of the new procedure were posted in drug storage areas and given to all staff members.
- The procedure was implemented. Charges were audited daily for 30 days. Results of the audit were reported to the QA Committee at the next meeting. Nonchargeable floor stock was reduced to $100, and there were only four drugs not charged directly to the patient to whom they had been administered.
- Random audits on ten surgery patients per month were conducted for the next six months. Average floor stock charges leveled off at about $30 per month, mostly in drugs and supplies not chargeable to the patient. In three of the six months, there were no drugs unaccounted for in the operating or recovery rooms.
- The QA Committee recommended that ten charts be audited monthly for charting accuracy, as an ongoing monitor.

Various problem-solving techniques were used to resolve the previously inaccurate floor stock charging procedure. Those involved in the delivery of the service helped design the improvements. Monitoring after implementation showed an improvement in service.

Some of the benefits of the above exercise are summarized below:

- Charges were recaptured and documented, resulting in an increase in revenue and a decrease in operating costs for both pharmacy and surgery.
- Patient care was improved because drugs were always on hand, and in date, when needed.
- Stock levels were reviewed and revised as needed. Insecurity of surgery personnel concerning availability of medications was alleviated.
- Costs of the assessment, reassessment, implementation, and in-service training were more than offset by the revenue generated by recapturing charges.
- The individuals involved had the satisfaction of working together to solve a problem and improve patient care.
- Tension between departments was reduced as the sources of past disagreements were eliminated.

As this case study demonstrates, the benefits of solving problems identified by quality assurance compensate for the time and expense to implement corrections. The solution is tailored to the problem. In addition, the problem remains corrected since monitoring mechanisms are built into the system.

WHAT TO DO IF THE PROBLEM IS NOT SOLVED

What if the results of reassessment indicate that the problem has not been corrected? It is advisable to review the initial assessment and decide whether:

- the problem was really correctable at the outset
- all the factors concerning the problem were correctly identified
- the corrective actions were appropriate
- the authority and responsibility were clearly and appropriately established for taking corrective actions
- corrective actions were actually carried out
- the sample size of the reassessment population was adequate to indicate that the problem still exists
- the reassessment measured the problem or its solution.[5]

If any of these decisions indicate that an error was made, it can be corrected and the reassessment can be repeated. A problem may seem to be uncorrectable when the real difficulty is based on resistance to change. It may be advisable to try reducing the severity of the problem initially, while decreasing resistance to change. Then, periodic reassessments should show progress toward improvement in the situation.

NOTES

1. A.C. Markus, "Quality Assurance—Panacea or Trojan Horse?" *Quality Review Bulletin,* February 1981, pp. 21-22.
2. Stanley A. Skillicorn, *Quality and Accountability* (San Francisco: Editorial Consultants, Inc., 1980), pp. 20-21.
3. K.O. Kaplan and J.M. Hopkins, *The QA Guide—A Resource for Hospital Quality Assurance* (Chicago: Joint Commission on Accreditation of Hospitals, 1980), pp. 119-124.
4. Skillicorn, *Quality and Accountability,* p. 31.
5. Kaplan and Hopkins, *The QA Guide,* pp. 126-127.

Chapter 5

Integrating Pharmacy's QA Program into the Hospital-Wide Plan

5

Regardless of which came first, the hospital's commitment to quality assurance or the pharmacy's QA activities, the functions of the pharmacy's QA plan must be integrated into the overall hospital plan. There are probably as many approaches to accomplishing this as there are methods of organizing the delivery of health care services in an institution.

THE QA PLAN FOR THE HOSPITAL

Since the Joint Commission on Accreditation of Hospitals (JCAH) requires only four standing hospital-wide committees (i.e., executive committee of governing body, executive committee of medical staff, infection control committee, and safety committee),[1] the other *functions* specified in the accreditation standards are often consolidated under the QA Committee. These activities include:

- planning
- identifying problems
- collecting and displaying data
- developing priorities for QA activities
- analyzing data
- suggesting improvement or changes
- taking corrective action
- monitoring results
- disseminating results
- reviewing and revising the QA program annually.

This list also can be used as a check to ensure that all required activities are carried out.[2]

The QA plan is a written reflection of the activities, responsibilities, and reporting systems actually in effect in the hospital. The following eleven guidelines should be considered before designing a hospital's QA plan:

1. State the purpose/goals/objectives of the QA program, remembering that the purpose is *not* to meet JCAH requirements.
2. Define the role of the key players (i.e., governing board, administrator, medical staff executive committee, medical staff, ancillary department).
3. Specify lines of authority, accountability, and communication.
4. Show how information is gathered and shared.
5. Review the hospital and medical staff's bylaws for purpose, structure, and authority statements. Be sure the design of the plan is in agreement with the bylaws. Tailor the plan to fit the type, size, and organizational structure of the hospital and scope of the services provided.
6. Report QA activities to a multidisciplinary group, as suggested by the following JCAH statement: "While the evaluation of physician-directed care must be performed by physician members of the medical staff, non-physician health care professionals should assess those aspects of care that they provide."[3]
7. Select an individual professional, administrator, member of the medical staff, or a committee to coordinate QA activities.
8. Organize the flow of information to maintain confidentiality.
9. Have the results of QA activities reported to the governing board. This not only gives support to QA activities but also permits follow-up on corrective actions.
10. Analyze QA activities, once each has been defined, to determine:
    - whether it should be conducted by an individual or a committee
    - at what level in the organization each activity should be performed.
11. Look for duplications of functions. The way to sell the program is to consolidate activities and reduce the number of committees in the hospital.[4]

The twelve elements to be included in the plan are:

1. statement of purpose—why is there a QA program?
2. goals and objectives—what will be accomplished?
3. scope of the program—who and what are involved?
4. organization plan—who will accomplish goals?
5. accountability—how will you know what is happening? To whom are QA activities reported?
6. implementation—how will the plan be carried out to accomplish objectives? Who has authority for taking action?

7. problem identification, prioritizing problems, assessing causes
8. development of measurable standards
9. selection of appropriate corrective actions
10. integration—do each department's QA activities mesh with hospital-wide plan?
11. supervision—is assessment/reassessment taking place when scheduled? Who is responsible for intervening when action is not taken, or when action is not effective?
12. evaluation—are problems being solved? Is patient care improving?[5]

Structural diagrams showing responsibility, authority, and accountability of committee organization can be drawn in many ways. For examples of various methods of organization, the reader is referred to the *QA Guide,* published by the JCAH.[6]

Analysis of various structural diagrams indicates that several factors appear to be required for success of the QA plan. For example:

- Separation of medical staff review from all other assessments provides confidentiality.
- A QA committee or coordinator reviews all surveys and refers them to the board of directors for action. Responses by the board are disseminated via the QA committee or coordinator.
- A multidisciplinary committee can best evaluate QA surveys and assess effectiveness or corrective action. Physicians must be involved in order to ensure cooperation from the medical staff.
- The QA Committee must have the authority to recommend corrective action, when necessary, but should not be responsible for carrying out the corrections. This should be done by the departments involved.[7]

Keeping medical staff performance evaluations separated from those of the nonmedical staff is one of the concepts that seems to be a vital component in the design of the plan. Two parallel groups, each ultimately reporting to the QA committee, can provide the functional structure that will carry out this concept. It may be helpful to keep a seesaw image in mind (Figure 5-1). In more formal terms this model could be represented as shown in Figure 5-2.

Several simple procedures make this system work. Based on the hospital bylaws, a decision-making group is appointed. It might be composed of the chief executive officer, the chief of staff, the director of nursing, one member of the governing body, and the QA coordinator. This group reports to the governing body directly and is responsible for setting priorities. The actual priorities for problem solving are established by the department directors close to the source of the

Figure 5-1 Neither Rides If Both Sides Don't Cooperate

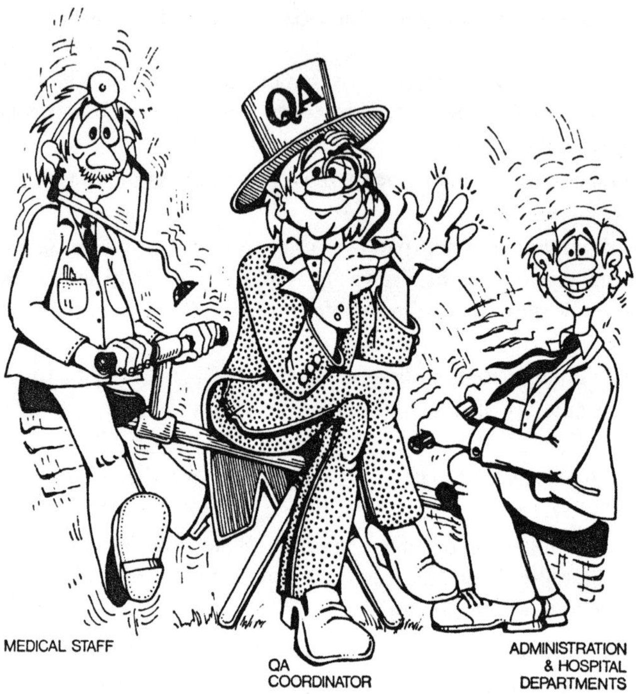

Figure 5-2 Proposed Organizational Structure for a Hospital's QA Committee

GOVERNING BOARD

JOINT CONFERENCE COMMITTEE

Medical Staff Executive Committee	Administrator
Chief of Staff	Department Directors
Medical Staff	Professional Departments

problem. Authority for decision making is given to the administrator (for professional departments) and the chief of staff (for the medical staff).

If an effective and efficient reporting system is designed, the hospital can expect to achieve many desirable goals. For example:

- Solutions can be facilitated closer to the source of the problem.
- Confidentiality of information can be maintained.
- Nonmedical staff problems are given the same amount of attention as medical staff problems.
- Two groups working simultaneously to solve problems can achieve more than one large group. Duplication of effort does not occur since different departments are represented within each group of the committee.
- Quality assurance becomes the center around which all quality-related activities revolve and from which improvements and the evaluation of care emanate.[8]

The JCAH is not insensitive to the political climate within a hospital, nor does it disregard the liability risks in establishing a QA program. The *QA Guide*, published by the JCAH, demonstrates this awareness in a list of attributes for a QA coordinator within the seven cautionary statements summarized below:[9]

1. The single most important attribute of the QA coordinator is that the individual must have the respect of both the medical and professional staff members of the hospital.
2. Communication and organizational skills are essential; it will be the coordinator's function to keep the committees moving toward solutions and to prevent them from bogging down in detail.
3. The coordinator needs to be able to understand and design management objectives and to understand and implement a "systems approach" to quality assurance.
4. Those involved in QA monitoring must be politically sensitive and aware of the need for confidentiality.
5. Since the QA coordinator usually serves a staff function (rather than a line function), he or she cannot enforce corrective action. However, the hospital administration and medical staff must demonstrate support for the authority of the QA coordinator.
6. If the coordinator is a member of the medical staff, the physician may not be interested in handling nonmedical staff problems.
7. The coordinator will have to help the committee decide the following:

- How are problems of medical staff versus those of nonmedical staff prioritized? Using the impact upon the patient as a criterion may lessen the sensitivity in this area.
- How are problems involving more than one department to be handled?
- How will all QA activities in the hospital be coordinated and integrated?
- Who has the authority for taking action?
- Who is responsible for intervening when the recommended actions are not taken or when the action taken is not effective?

Another option for designing the structure of QA activities that should be mentioned is that of sharing the functions with one or more hospitals or between like departments in various institutions. This has worked successfully for hospitals in a geographical region that have the same medical staff members. The Eastern Michigan Region of the Sisters of Mercy Health Corporation designed a hospital pharmacy QA program to be implemented in seven of their hospitals.[10] All of the pharmacies in the HPI Hospital Pharmacies, Inc., management group use the identical QA format that is integrated into each respective hospital's QA plan.[11] By comparing results with similar institutions, it is possible to judge performance and expand the data base beyond one's own limited area.

THE QUALITY CIRCLE CONCEPT

The concept of the quality circle developed in the United States in the 1940s. After World War II, Japan adopted it as a method to improve the technology and quality of its products. While Japan was implementing the method, the United States slowly discontinued its use. However, with the dynamic impact that Japanese products have had on the marketplace, many American industries have reinstated quality circles. Recent trends indicate that there is a place in health care for this concept as well.[12]

Simply stated, a quality circle has the following characteristics:

- It is a group composed of individuals from all levels of technical and management activities.
- Membership in the group is voluntary.
- The group leader (or facilitator) does not participate in decision making.
- The group collects data, identifies problems, suggests improvements, and reports its recommendations to management.

It is very efficient to allow employees to find solutions to their own problems. They are close to the problems and can quickly determine whether proposed remedies will be feasible. The quality circle in St. Agnes Hospital in Fond du Lac, Wisconsin, has been formed to improve patient care, communications, morale and job satisfaction, cost containment, and efficiency.[13] There is also a QA program at the hospital.

In order for the system to work, management must be willing to listen to the recommendations submitted by the group and to evaluate them objectively. The concept of quality circles is a formalized structure for problem identification that could become an integral part of future QA programs in hospitals.

MULTIDISCIPLINARY ACTIVITIES—AN ILLUSTRATION

One of the strongest arguments supporting quality assurance in hospital pharmacy is that it requires interaction with others on the health care team. In fact, the JCAH standard states, "while the evaluation of physician-directed care must be performed by physician members of the medical staff, non-physician health care members should assess those aspects of care that they provide."[14]

With the increase in emphasis on clinical pharmacy services in the past several years, the astute hospital pharmacist can use quality assurance to justify the need for these activities. The two functions dovetail perfectly: quality assurance identifies a problem; clinical pharmacy solves it. Quality assurance then assures administration that the problem is solved, the solution, effective.

To use the guidelines stated earlier for QA programs, two recently published articles will be discussed concerning the incidence of drug-induced illnesses in hospitalized patients.

Steel and associates conducted a study on 815 patients on two medical nursing units in a university hospital.[15] For the purpose of the study, the authors defined iatrogenic illness as any illness that resulted from a diagnostic procedure, from any form of therapy, or from any harmful occurrences that are not natural consequences of the patient's disease. They found that 209 patients had a drug-related complication and that of all patient complications, 53 percent had at least one problem related to exposure to a drug. Therefore, despite the conservative design of the experiment, the authors demonstrated a positive correlation between drug exposure and the development of a complication. This was corroborated by the observation that those patients who developed no complications received fewer drugs during the entire hospital stay, as compared with the number of drugs prescribed for patients who later developed complications. The authors describe a need for new methods of monitoring patients: "mechanisms must be developed to assess the hazards of hospitalization in an ongoing manner."

Myers, in an editorial in the same issue of the *New England Journal of Medicine,* suggests a method for conducting this monitoring using computers.[16] Zellmer, in an editorial in the May 1981 issue of the *American Journal of Hospital Pharmacy,* reflects the fact that neither of these articles mentions the role that the pharmacist could play in monitoring and preventing such drug-induced, adverse effects.[17]

Using this evidence as background, a hospital pharmacist can review the incidence of similar complications occurring in his or her own institution. This may be difficult to do, because documentation is generally vague. In addition, the inherent liability in such situations reduces the availability of information even further. However, if research *does* reveal the potential for such a problem, the opportunity for a multidisciplinary QA activity exists.

Medical staff, nursing, pharmacy, and medical records personnel are all involved in the functions of prescribing, dispensing, administering, and recording medications. If an adverse effect does take place, risk management and hospital administration may also become involved. Using the previously stated principles, those who provide the service should be involved in monitoring and improving it. The results of assessment and reassessment audits should be reported to the QA committee for analysis, recommendation, and action.

By searching for similar research opportunities in the hospital, the pharmacist can gain entrance into patient monitoring functions that encompass several disciplines. Participation in this type of group allows the pharmacist to demonstrate effectiveness, improve clinical therapy, fulfill requirements for QA activities, and work as a peer with other health care professionals.

ROLES OF THE KEY PLAYERS

Earlier in this chapter, specific functions were assigned to certain individuals. The roles played by these people are derived from the hospital bylaws and the QA plan. A summary of these key players and the scope of each role are provided below:[18]

Governing body:

- "It is the governing body's responsibility to establish, maintain and support, through the hospital's administration and medical staff, an ongoing QA Program."[19]

Hospital administration (chief executive officer):

- shares delegated responsibility for the program with medical staff
- is accountable for activities involving professional and ancillary departments
- is the liaison with medical staff via medical staff executive committee.

Chief medical officer:

- shares delegated responsibility with administration for the program
- is accountable for activities involving medical staff
- acts as liaison with professional and ancillary departments via QA or joint conference committee
- coordinates peer review activities.

Each clinical practitioner:

- is responsible for identifying and resolving problems related to care each provides. Reports to chief of medical staff.

Department directors:

- are responsible for identifying and resolving problems involving each respective department
- report to administrator via QA committee
- participate in hospital-wide QA plan.

QA coordinator:

- organizes and coordinates all QA activities
- collects, collates, and displays data and results of audits
- refers items to medical executive committee, administration, governing board, or respective hospital departments, as necessary
- keeps records and ensures that all QA activities take place at the scheduled times
- monitors performance of corrective actions.

It is essential that neither the QA coordinator nor the hospital administrator be responsible for carrying out corrective actions. Their function is to ensure that the appropriate corrective actions are taken.

If a positive attitude can be maintained by all the players, the logical conclusion of the "QA scenario" will be a "happy ending": the improvement of patient care in the hospital.

NOTES

1. *Accreditation Manual for Hospitals* (Chicago: Joint Commission on Accreditation of Hospitals, 1981), pp. 105-109.
2. Karen O. Kaplan and Julie M. Hopkins, *The QA Guide–A Resource for Hospital Quality Assurance* (Chicago: Joint Commission on Accreditation of Hospitals, 1980), pp. 20-21.
3. *Accreditation Manual for Hospitals,* pp. 151-154.
4. Kaplan and Hopkins, *QA Guide,* pp. 38-39.
5. Dianne Moeller, "Hospital-Wide Quality Assurance—A Management Perspective," Association of Western Hospitals Seminar, Anaheim, California, April 28, 1981.
6. Kaplan and Hopkins, *QA Guide,* pp. 27-36.
7. Ibid., pp. 21-32.
8. Robert Redman, ed., "Symposia Supports Philosophy of Quality Assurance Standard," *Perspectives,* May/June 1981, pp. 9-10.
9. Kaplan and Hopkins, *QA Guide,* pp. 21-32.
10. Richard Hoffman et al., "Development of a Multi-Hospital Pharmacy Quality Assurance Program," *Hospital Pharmacy* 15 (1980): 365-380.
11. Kenneth N. Horowitz and Marlene Lamnin, "Design and Implementation of a Quality Assurance Program for Pharmaceutical Services," *American Journal of Hospital Pharmacy* 37 (January 1980): 82-84.
12. "Hospital Quality Circles Improve Quality and Productivity," *Hospital Peer Review* 6, no. 9 (1981): 101-103.
13. Ibid.
14. *Accreditation Manual for Hospitals,* pp. 151-154.
15. Knight Steel et al., "Iatrogenic Illness on a General Medical Service at a University Hospital," *New England Journal of Medicine* 304, no. 11 (1981): 638-642.
16. Jack D. Myers, "Preventing Iatrogenic Complications," *New England Journal of Medicine* 304, no. 11 (1981): 664-665.
17. William A. Zellmer, "Can Pharmacists Prevent Drug-Induced Illness in Hospitals?" *American Journal of Hospital Pharmacy 38* no. 5 (1981): 637.
18. *Accreditation Manual for Hospitals,* p. 151.
19. Ibid.

Part II

Pharmacy-Specific Quality Assurance

Chapter 6

Purchasing and Inventory Control

6

Buying a cheap article to save money is like stopping a clock to save time.
—Anonymous

The traditional role of the pharmacist, whether in community practice or in an institution, is based on the effect of the medications prescribed, dispensed, and administered to the patient. It follows, then, that the level of quality of the services provided can be no better than the quality of the pharmaceutical products involved. At the foundation of this premise is the trust placed in the skill and knowledge of the pharmacist, by the patients, for selection of appropriate medications. Moreover, when the choice of specific brands or generics is left to the discretion of the pharmacist, the responsibility is even greater: the liability for the incorrect choice will rest entirely upon the pharmacist. Clearly, the subject of quality assurance for purchasing and inventory control is one of the key issues facing practitioners. Therefore, the pharmacy-specific section of this text begins with these controls.

VENDOR APPROVAL PROCEDURES

The 1970s was a decade of transition in the pharmaceutical industry: antisubstitution laws were repealed, thus allowing more freedom of choice for the consumer and the pharmacist in the selection of products.[1] The "Drug Product Quality Statement," issued in 1970 by the Academy of Pharmaceutical Sciences of the American Pharmaceutical Association (APhA), defines the characteristics a pharmacist should look for when selecting a product.[2] Samples of the types of items that could be included in vendor evaluation procedures are listed in Exhibit 6-1.

Exhibit 6-1 Information Request for Vendor Evaluation

1. Copy of current liability insurance coverage.
2. List of recalls (and reason for recall) over last three years.
3. Copy of FDA inspection reports (Form 483) for last three years, and responses by company to any deficiencies.
4. Complete list of products and prices, indicating original supplier, if items are manufactured by another source.
5. Copies of NDA or ANDA approval letters for applicable products.
6. Copies of bioavailability studies on applicable products.
7. Copies of stability studies for products, especially those in unit dose packaging.
8. Pictures of facilities.
9. Permission for the evaluator to tour facility.
10. Sterility test results where applicable; also results of other tests, where applicable, e.g., content uniformity, dissolution, etc.
11. Return goods policy.
12. Willingness to bid.
13. Willingness to reimburse customer for price difference from alternate source, if vendor unable to supply bid/price protected products at agreed upon price.
14. Ability to supply if sales increase.
15. Participation in group purchasing and prime vendor contracts.
16. List of shortages or inability to supply (for 30 days or more) over last two years.
17. Availability of educational materials and product information from company. List of speakers available for in-hospital seminars.
18. Sample labels (and/or product samples, including labeling) for products.

Exhibit 6-1 continued

19. Assurance that the company will guarantee that products shipped will have no less than one-year shelf life.
20. Method of shipping used. Required minimum order quantity or minimum dollar amount. Shipping costs are prepaid if purchases are over minimum quantity.
21. Sample package inserts.

Legally, the pharmacist is responsible for ensuring that drugs dispensed by the pharmacy are safe and effective. Moreover, cost containment efforts require that drugs be economical. To provide these guarantees, the pharmacist must review the quality of products and services provided by various outside sources. Therefore, before beginning formulary limitation, the pharmacist must also check state laws for specifications concerning therapeutic equivalency.

With the myriad of generic products available, as well as several sources for most trade name products, the pharmacist must reduce the number of sources of supply to keep down the "costs of doing business." Medicare and other fiscal intermediaries also require proof that "prudent buying" procedures are being used. This means that if a hospital purchases a drug that is not at the lowest cost available, an explanation must be provided for the purchasing decision that was made. However, if Medicare does not accept the explanation, it can disallow the difference between the lowest cost and that price that the hospital paid.[3] In the latter situation, the financial impact could be astronomical.

Fortunately, there are many sources of information that the pharmacist can turn to for guides on vendor selection. Of these, two excellent references are the "Guidelines for Selecting Pharmaceutical Manufacturers and Distributors," from the American Society of Hospital Pharmacists (ASHP)[4] and "The Assessment of Vendors of Multisource Drug Products by the Pharmacist," published by the School of Pharmacy of the University of North Carolina at Chapel Hill.[5]

As each vendor is reviewed, it is advisable to document the reasons for approval or rejection of each company. A list of approved vendors is compiled and annually reviewed for appropriateness. As new product or service lines are added, vendors may also be reevaluated. Assurance that all purchases are made only from approved vendors is the foundation for QA activities in inventory control. At a scheduled interval (e.g., once a month), pharmacists should also review invoices and outstanding purchase orders to spot-check for nonapproved vendors or for sources other than the primary supplier.

The Joint Commission on Accreditation of Hospitals (JCAH) requires that the hospital's Pharmacy and Therapeutics Committee (or its equivalent) annually approve both the purchasing services and the formulary.[6] It is also necessary to have a mechanism for notifying all medical and nursing staff members of additions or deletions to the formulary.

There are many sources of information available to the pharmacist responsible for making these purchasing decisions. One place to turn for help is the local or regional buying group. The group or individual decision maker(s) will have screened many potential vendors and may have even conducted plant inspections. Purchasing agents for government agencies, such as county or state facilities, may also have these types of data. The options open to those individuals responsible for making purchasing decisions include:

- buying direct from the manufacturer, using bid or contract pricing when feasible
- participating in a buying group
- buying from the wholesaler, with or without "prime vendor" services
- Any combination of the above.

Each method has its merits, and each should be considered as a possible method of purchasing from every vendor with whom the pharmacy is doing business.

The trend in obtaining drugs and supplies for hospitals has shifted in the past several years toward group purchasing. By pooling efforts to select sources and products, hospitals increase their buying "clout" with their suppliers. The prudent purchasing agent or pharmacist must select the group as carefully as he or she would choose vendors. If a buying group has a reputation for compliance with bid purchasing contracts, better prices will be offered to the group the following year. If a group accepts bids from competitors, there will be an incentive to "cherry pick" the best prices from each source, a practice that decreases the credibility of the group's dedication to its contracts.

It is conceivable that an individual hospital could obtain better prices by dealing with the manufacturer personally, rather than by participating in a buying group. If the institution is very large or has a prestigious reputation, or if the buying group is known for a low level of compliance to its bids, the hospital may be able to achieve better contracts on its own. One way to establish whether the bid group actually achieves better bids is to compare the prices quoted single hospitals in the geographical area with those offered to the group.

The FDA maintains information on vendors that is available to the public through the Freedom of Information Office. Material on a specific company may be obtained by writing to the FDA office having jurisdiction over the specific geographical location of the vendor.

Replies will be "purged" of confidential information before release by the FDA. Some of the material available from this source is listed below.

- records of recalls
- findings upon plant inspection (form 483) and responses by the company to these reports
- analysis of field samples of products obtained by FDA inspectors
- NDA and ANDA approvals
- regulatory letters by the FDA and responses by the company

A time period for the required information from the FDA (e.g., the past two years) should be specified. There is a charge for photocopy costs exceeding five dollars.

In 1972, the ASHP adopted an advertising policy for its journal in which the Society reserved the right to have an ASHP representative conduct an on-site review of facilities before approving advertisements from a new company.[7] Therefore, those vendors whose advertisements appear in the American Journal of Hospital Pharmacy have already undergone preliminary screening by the Society. The company may not use this endorsement in any of its literature, however.

Most manufacturers are happy to provide pharmacists with any information that leads to approved vendor status. Any company that refuses to provide information, or to permit a tour of facilities, does not deserve to be approved. The pharmacist cannot make an intelligent decision on product selection unless all the facts are available.

There is one caveat that the purchaser must consider: many companies are distributors or relabelers; they do not manufacture their own products. It is essential to trace the source of drugs back to the manufacturer. *Both* the name of the manufacturer *and* the distributor should be printed on the label. It is essential that the pharmacist receive a written assurance that notification will be sent if the source of a particular drug is changed.

LIMITING THE INVENTORY: THERAPEUTIC SUBSTITUTION

The benefits of a QA program in the pharmacy can really be demonstrated in this area, in a language easily understood by administration—that of dollars and cents.

Monitoring prescribing habits, by means of computer utilization reports and drug utilization reviews, reveals duplications of inventory products. A utilization review can focus on specific disease entities and suggest reductions in the formulary. Not only will there be an immediate realization in terms of credit for returned drugs, but there will also be other benefits.[8] Reduction of assets tied up in inventory is a real achievement. Since fewer products and sources are used, buying procedures become more efficient, reducing the cost of handling purchase orders and invoices. Predicting usage of specific drug entities becomes more reliable, thus increasing credibility with vendors. This leads to better prices and bids for the hospital and lower costs for the patient.

Two cases from the literature demonstrate the value of limiting inventory: One example of savings achieved by therapeutic substitution took place at the Veterans Administration Hospital in Buffalo, New York.[9] An average of $3.50 per prescription was saved when the pharmacist called the physician and suggested prescribing generic products or one of the usually stocked brand names instead. The overall savings accrued over 250 workdays was $5,821.77. Another hospital reported that savings achieved by formulary limitations in just one class of drugs, theophyllines, was reported to be $16,301.71 in one year.[10] By extrapolating such savings to other categories of drugs, such as antibiotics, one can easily justify the time spent on these efforts.

The Pharmacy and Therapeutics Committee has the ultimate authority to approve or reject products for the formulary. Some hospitals develop a mechanism for a physician's request of a nonformulary drug for a particular patient and condition.[11] It is not the intent of the pharmacy to prevent a patient from receiving the special care required; rather, the formulary is designed to recognize the exceptional situation, as contrasted to those of the majority of patients, who will achieve the desired therapeutic goals with the usually stocked items.

After implementing therapeutic substitution, an analysis of the number of orders actually filled for nonformulary drugs is conducted during a specific time period. This will indicate whether any drugs should be considered for addition to the formulary. Conversely, lack of utilization of formulary drugs may indicate an opportunity for a deletion from inventory.

The need for educating specific members of the medical staff may also be detected in this way. Trends and patterns in nosocomial (hospital-acquired) and community infections must be monitored and compared with the sensitivity of the drugs being prescribed. This comparison provides an opportunity for pharmacists to work with the clinical laboratory staff to ensure appropriate therapy.

One additional benefit may also be possible. Limiting the number of drugs in any category reduces the potential for drug error. This is certainly a goal to strive for and another strong justification for the program.

COMPLIANCE TO BID PROGRAMS

Once bids have been awarded and contracts are in effect, it is easier to establish controls to foster adherence to bid purchasing. On the buying end, the process begins with the education of those who are purchasing drugs from the various primary sources. Complete alphabetical listing of drugs, with primary source of supply and prices, along with inventory or "buy" cards containing pertinent bid and contract information, will also enhance and encourage this process.

A review of purchase orders can be conducted periodically and an exception report prepared, listing those items that fail to comply with bid contracts. A similar review of invoices and a report of exceptions can also be prepared. Analysis of both reports can reveal sources of problems, leading to noncompliance in purchasing practices. Since the benefits for compliance can be documented in real dollars, it is easier to motivate employees to follow these established procedures.

On the receiving end, procedures can be devised to check all invoices for correct pricing and discounts, before marking merchandise. If those employees conducting receiving activities are trained to place into stock only those items that have been verified and labeled, unmarked or incorrectly marked items will not appear in any area of the department of the hospital. Periodic checks on each section of inventory can monitor this procedure. There is an added benefit in that less activity will be required to prepare the department for scheduled inventory procedures.

There is always a temptation to order needed items from the wholesaler. When using the prime vendor concept of purchasing, this presents no problem. The prime vendor concept is a method used to reduce acquisition costs by centralizing purchases from many vendors, into one "prime" vendor. For example, a drug wholesaler carries tablets, capsules, liquids, and injectables from many major manufacturers and sells them at their invoice cost, plus a fee, to the hospitals. Reducing the amount of time spent processing purchase orders, invoices, and credit vouchers also reduces the cost of conducting purchasing procedures. The benefits of direct buying, plus the convenience of receiving a shipment from a local wholesaler, are combined in a single source. However, stock levels can be maintained, since the time lag created by buying from the manufacturer has been eliminated.

In order for the prime vendor concept to function efficiently, both the wholesaler and the purchasing group or pharmacy must agree to abide by specific commitments. The supplier must be willing to provide:

- a full range of product sizes, strengths, and dosage forms
- computerized utilization and management reports
- efficient delivery systems, including emergency service

- responsive, experienced sales representatives
- a complete program of products and services.

On the other hand, the purchaser also has specific obligations to fulfill. The hospital, or group, must deliver:

- a total commitment to the program
- prompt payment
- a skilled inventory manager to work with the supplier
- ability and willingness to respond to computerized reports
- participation in only one buying group
- fulfillment of projected purchasing quantities.

When Riverside Methodist Hospital in Columbus, Ohio (a 923-bed facility), implemented prime vendor buying methods, some impressive savings were achieved:[12]

- Inventory turnover rate doubled, from 5.9 to 13.4 turns per year.
- Inventory was reduced 56 percent, from $392,000 to $171,000 (excluding intravenous solutions).
- The staff required to handle purchasing functions was reduced by 1.4 full-time equivalents.
- Accounting costs were reduced by $24,000.
- The acquisition costs of drugs decreased by 6.8 percent.
- The number of sources for pharmacy items was reduced from 60 to 10 vendors.
- The cash flow difference in the first year of operation was $466,000.

By prorating these figures to compensate for differences in hospital size, one can determine the dramatic impact that prime vendor purchasing can produce.

Even greater savings can be achieved if the wholesaler and supplier consent to abide by contracts or bid prices negotiated with the hospital as a three-way agreement. If not on prime vendor purchasing, however, wholesaler invoices should be monitored for bid items, indicating potential short supply or slow delivery situations. This is a valuable tool for the purchasing manager.

If a computer is available to the pharmacy, internal reports can be generated for utilization of specific drugs, for the number of inventory turns, for the amount of purchases and discounts from each vendor, and for many other valuable pieces of information. Controls built into the system, using computer printouts as data sources, are valuable parts of the QA program. Comparison of actual results to preestablished standards provide a readily available monitoring device.

MONITORING OUTDATES

Both JCAH and Medicare require that all drug storage areas be checked once a month by pharmacy personnel.[13,14] This includes crash carts, floor stock, night locker, ancillary departments, and any area where drugs are stored outside the pharmacy. As part of this procedure, the pharmacy staff can rotate stock, so that short-dated items are in the main pharmacy, where they are more likely to be used. The name of the next expiring drug and its expiration date should be posted on the outside of the crash cart. This is another area where the QA program can ensure compliance.

Various systems have been devised to control, identify, isolate, and return expiring drugs:

- assigning a color to each month or year. As each month approaches, the expiring items are identified and removed from stock.
- circling the expiration date with a colored felt-tipped pen if date will occur within the present calendar year
- entering expiration dates in a log as every drug is received
- keeping a chart for each crash cart, indicating the expiration date of every item in the cart.

Documentation for nursing unit and ancillary department stock is usually inspected by JCAH and Medicare auditors. Therefore, it is vital to document these checking procedures and keep them up to date.

The JCAH standards concerning storage of pharmaceuticals should be reviewed. The pharmacist can prepare a checklist of these items, to ensure that each is monitored every month. One such list should be filled out every month for each unit, and the date of the inspection and name of the individual conducting the inspection should be recorded. It is recommended that a nurse co-sign the list after the inspection, so that documentation exists for initiating any necessary corrective action. Refrigerators used to store medications must be monitored daily, the temperature recorded, and adjustments made if the temperature varies from predetermined levels.

Those items that can be returned for credit must be removed from stock and set aside in a specially designated area to prevent accidental dispensing of these items. It is also advisable to prepare a medication destruction record to document the disposal of drugs that are not returnable. The signature of a pharmacist and a witness should appear on this record, especially when controlled substances (Schedules II through V) are involved. The state regulations for controlled substances must be checked along with the method of proper disposal or return of Schedule II drugs. Also included in the list of drugs to be destroyed, with documentation, are any expired drugs packaged by the pharmacy and any personal patient medications kept in the pharmacy after patient dismissal from the hospital. Personal patient medications are usually kept 30 to 60 days, then destroyed, if not claimed by the patient or family.

One of the basic responsibilities of a pharmacist is to ensure that medications dispensed to patients are effective. Therefore, there is a continuous need for pharmacy employees to remove expired medications from active stock and to ensure that drugs are stored correctly. QA mechanisms can be established to safeguard the potency of the pharmacy inventory.

RECORD KEEPING

Natural progression from the information presented in the previous section leads to all of the requirements for keeping records. Regarding the length of time various items are to be stored, there are two general rules:

1. Check state and federal regulations: the longer time period takes precedence; for example, if the state law requires that a record be kept three years, and the federal law only two, the longer time period (three years for the state) applies.
2. Documentation required by JCAH should be kept for the interval between inspections; that is, if a two-year accreditation was achieved after the last inspection, then the pharmacy will be responsible for two years' worth of documentation on the next inspection.

Records may also be stored in a computer. State and federal regulations should be checked for specific requirements. Since storage space is always at a premium, it is advisable to review the records in storage, at least annually, and to discard those no longer required. Building these checks and reviews into the QA assessment process ensures:

- a readily retrievable audit trail
- removal of unnecessary records in a timely manner
- a periodic check that documents are stored properly (i.e., safely and accessibly).

Examples of the types of records required for purchasing and inventory control are listed in Exhibit 6-2.

Exhibit 6-2 Required Purchasing and Inventory Control Records

I. Controlled Substances

- DEA order blanks
- Purchase orders (Schedule II purchases filed separately)
- Invoices
- Biannual inventory
- Perpetual inventory records
- Dispensing records, e.g., floor stock control sheets
- Returns of outdated drugs
- Destruction of outdated drugs
- Prescription files
- Reports of missing or stolen drugs
- Staff physicians' DEA numbers and signatures
- Current state and federal licenses

II. Purchasing and Other Records

- Purchase orders and record of use of each purchase order number
- Record of credits outstanding from vendors
- Inventory records
- Drug defects reported to FDA
- Drug recalls and record of how each was handled
- Unit dose packaging records
- Manufacturing log, if applicable
- Record of warrantees, guarantees and service contracts on equipment

DRUG RECALLS

Drug recall information is sent to the hospital pharmacist in many forms:

- letters from the FDA or the manufacturer announcing a recall
- weekly newsletter from the FDA (formerly free, now available by subscription at $45/year)[15]
- recall sections in various newsletters from professional organizations (e.g., ASHP and APhA)
- reprint information: some wholesalers reprint and supply recall information to their customers as a professional service.

It is necessary to document that a thorough search was made for any drug involved in a recall. This can be done simply by writing the date, the name of the pharmacist, and the results of the search for the drug on the recall letter. Disposal of any stock should also be recorded. A more elaborate system involves preparation of a form listing the drug name and strength, date and reason for recall, name of manufacturer or distributor, and every area in the hospital where the drug might be found. A sample of this type of documentation is shown in Exhibit 6-3.

If necessary, it is important, in the event of a recall, to have a policy covering the handling of notification of medical staff, nursing, pharmacy and therapeutics committee, and patients. Furthermore, when a recall results in a short supply of a drug, the nursing and medical staff should be alerted.

An annual review of recall records could uncover potential problems with a vendor. This review helps convert a tiresome record-keeping activity into a meaningful part of the purchasing and inventory control QA program. Sample standards for measuring the effectiveness of the purchasing and inventory control activities in the pharmacy are presented in Exhibit 6-4.

MATERIEL MANAGEMENT

Efficient management of sterile and nonsterile supplies in a hospital is a process vital to the day-to-day functioning of the institution. In some facilities the director of pharmacy is also the materiel manager. In others the pharmacy department is one component of the materiel management service. Regardless of the reporting mechanism the two functions are intimately related. The subject is mentioned briefly here because of the current trend in hospitals to relate the two activities to each other.

Exhibit 6-3 Drug Recall Record

Date__________________

Drug Name______________________ Strength____________ Size_______

Manufacturer or Distributor______________________________________

Reason for Recall____

Class of Recall (I, II or III) _____________

AREAS CHECKED	AMOUNT FOUND	DATE	INITIALS
Nursing Units			
1.			
2.			
3.			
4.			
5.			
Night Locker			
Emergency Room			
OR/RR/Delivery Room			
Clinic			
Pharmacy - active stock			
Pharmacy - unit dose stock			
Pharmacy - back-up stock			
Pharmacy - expired drugs waiting for return			
Medication Carts			
Crash Carts			
Outpatient Prescription Records			

Disposal Method:____

Date:_____________________

Signature of Pharmacist:____

Exhibit 6-4 QA Standards for Purchasing and Inventory Control

1. No medications shall be ordered from vendors not on Approved Vendor List.
2. There shall be no medications stocked, dispensed or administered that are outdated.
3. There shall be no mislabeled, adulterated or misbranded products on the shelf, or within the hospital.
4. All returns shall be processed at least quarterly (two of these to coincide with semi-annual inventory).
5. There shall be no medications in stock for administration or dispensing that have been recalled.
6. All controlled substances shall have records of acquisition and disposition readily available.
7. Date of purchase, acquisition cost and vendor must be identifiable for all stock.
8. All medications on bid are purchased from a vendor with contract (except where documentation within hospital exists for deviation).

Source: Quality Assurance Program, HPI Hospital Pharmacies, Inc., © 1979. Reprinted with permission.

Both process and outcome standards are necessary for measuring the quality of services in materiel management because of the varied types of functions performed in the department. Activities such as decontamination, processing, and sterilizing can be measured using process standards to ensure that department procedures are carefully followed. Purchasing and charging procedures, however, lend themselves to process or outcome assessment or both.

To design standards in order to measure performance in materiel management, the same process described earlier for analyzing and monitoring pharmacy activities is used:

- define quality
- write standards
- assess performance
- identify problems
- take corrective action
- reassess performance
- redefine quality.

To find and identify problems in the materiel management realm, a "problem log" may be of value. Such a record was described at a seminar for operating room and central service supervisors held in New York City in 1981.[16] Problems recognized within the department, as well as complaints from other departments or patients, are recorded in the log in chronological order. The log permits entries for actions and results for each problem. After the problem has been identified, it is transcribed onto a six-step QA form, which includes the following data:

1. nature of the problem and when reported to QA department
2. how problem was found
3. investigation conducted
4. actions taken
5. results of corrective actions
6. findings at follow-up.

This same type of device could be used in any department of the hospital to collect problems and report progress toward their correction.

There are many references that can be used as guides to develop a materiel management QA program. It is not within the scope of this book to detail how to establish a QA program for materiel management; however, a list of areas suggested for inclusion in such a program is presented below as a starting point. The methodology is the same for all hospital departments.

- purchasing and inventory control
- decontamination
- processing
- sterilization
- storage
- infection control
- distribution
- charging

- department management
- policies and procedures manuals
- record keeping
- maintenance of equipment.

A review of guidelines published by the Center for Disease Control and JCAH will provide most of the information required to write standards in this field.

The presence of some services in materiel management varies with the organization of the hospital (e.g., print shop, transportation, food service). These departments would also require QA monitoring, tailored to the specific functions in each area.

It is possible to design an objective, quantifiable QA program with point values assigned to various activities. Then each employee will know the goal to be attained, and all employees can be measured by the same rating scale. An example of this type of program is explained in the January-February 1980 issue of *Hospital Topics*.[17] Some cautions to be observed with this type of assessment include the following:

- A random sample of department activities is used to assess performance. The items in the sample must be carefully selected to give an overall, valid picture of the department's functions.
- Scoring the assessments of an individual's performance and contrasting the results to those of his or her peers can be a demotivator. However, it can also be an effective management tool in the hands of a strong manager, one who can also deemphasize the negative results.

The General Accounting Office (GAO) report published in 1979 describes purchasing and materiel management functions in private hospitals.[18] Part II of this report includes a checklist for evaluating various functions within the sphere of purchasing and materiel management. The pharmacist should modify this checklist to meet the needs of the institution, but it is an effective and comprehensive guide for establishing QA standards.

CONCLUSION

The current trend in hospital pharmacy is leading the pharmacist away from purely distributive functions and toward more patient-centered clinical activities. In order for this transition to occur, however, all systems in the pharmacy must be running smoothly. QA activities, therefore, provide a mechanism whereby the controls built into all pharmacy systems are maintained.

In addition, quality assurance in purchasing and inventory control demonstrates the competency of the pharmacist to select appropriate, economical therapeutic agents. Once the basic skills of pharmacy are accepted by the nursing and medical staff, the pharmacist can build on this trust to expand into other clinical areas.

NOTES

1. Virginia Bates Johnson, "Drug Product Selection Through the Decades," *American Pharmacy* NS20, no. 10 (1980): 572-576.

2. "Drug Product Quality Statement," *Journal of the American Pharmaceutical Association* NS10 (1980): 107.

3. Robert L. Janson, *Purchasing Agent's Desk Book* (Englewood Cliffs, N.J.: Prentice-Hall, 1980), p. 197.

4. "ASHP Guidelines for Selecting Pharmaceutical Manufacturers and Distributors," *American Journal of Hospital Pharmacy* 35 (November 1977): 1252-1253.

5. Robert W. Ritter et al., *The Assessment of Vendors of Multisource Drug Products by the Pharmacist* (Chapel Hill, N.C.: North Carolina Pharmaceutical Research Foundation, 1979).

6. *Accreditation Manual for Hospitals* (Chicago: Joint Commission on Accreditation of Hospitals, 1980), pp. 137-145.

7. "ASHP Policy on Advertising," *American Journal of Hospital Pharmacy*, November 1977, pp. 1252-1253.

8. Jack McPartland, "Alternative Medication for Outpatients Provides Savings," *Hospital Pharmacy* 15 (1980): 424-425.

9. Ibid.

10. J.V. Anandan, "Reducing the Number of Formulary Theophylline Preparations," *American Journal of Hospital Pharmacy* 38 (1981): 511-513.

11. Normand A. Pelissier et al., "Physician's Antibiotic Order Form," letter, *Hospital Pharmacy* 14 (1980): 425.

12. Thomas Sherrin, *Wholesaler Servicing of Hospitals* (videotape) (Scarsdale, N.Y.: National Wholesale Druggists Association, 1981).

13. *Accreditation Manual for Hospitals*, pp. 137-145.

14. "Conditions for Participation," Medicare Regulations, Department of Health, Education and Welfare, Washington, D.C., 1969, publications no. 19,821, Reg. Sec. 405.1027, #b2.

15. *FDA Enforcement Report* (Rockville, Md.: Food and Drug Administration, 1981).

16. "Central Service and Operating Room Supervisors Gather for Quality Assurance Seminar," *Hospital Purchasing News* 5, no. 9 (1981): 12.

17. Robert C. Richardson, "A Quality Control Program for Central Supply, " *Hospital Topics*, January/February 1980.

18. U.S. General Accounting Office, *Study of Purchasing and Materials Management Functions in Private Hospitals: Opportunities for Improving Hospital Purchasing, Inventory Management and Supply Distribution*, Part I (PSAD-79-58A) and Part II (PSAD-79-58B) (Washington, D.C.: General Accounting Office, April 1979).

SUGGESTED READINGS

Approved Prescription Drug Products with Therapeutic Equivalence Evaluation. U.S. Department of Health and Human Services, Food and Drug Administration, Washington, D.C.: U.S. Government Printing Office, 1981.

The Bioavailability of Drug Products, cumulative edition. Washington, D.C.: American Pharmaceutical Association, 1978.

Checklist and Guidelines for Evaluating Purchasing and Materiel Management Functions in Private Hospitals, Parts I and II. Washington, D.C.: U.S. Government Printing Office, 1979, publication no. 0-620-167/271.

Dittert, Lewis, W., and Dianta, Anthony R. "The Bioavailability of Drug Products." *Journal of the American Pharmaceutical Association* NS13(8) (1973): 421-432.

Housley, Charles E. *Hospital Materiel Management.* Rockville, Md.: Aspen Systems Corporation, 1978.

Johnson, Richard E.; Campbell, William H.; and Christensen, Dale N. "Quality Assurance of Pharmaceutical Services in Hospitals." *American Journal of Hospital Pharmacy* 31(1974): 640-647.

Lamy, P.P., and Flack, H.L. "A Plant Survey Form for Evaluating Pharmaceutical Quality Control." *American Journal of Hospital Pharmacy* 25 (1968): 183-189.

A Manual for Hospital Central Services. Washington, D.C.: Department of Health, Education and Welfare Publication, publication no. 017-022-00387-2, April 1975.

Multisource Drug Products Derived from the Drug Products Information File. Washington, D.C.: American Society of Hospital Pharmacists, 1976.

Ritter, Robert W. et al. *The Assessment of Vendors of Multisource Drug Products by the Pharmacist.* Chapel Hill, N.C.: North Carolina Pharmaceutical Research Foundation, 1979.

Sanderson, Edward D. *Hospital Purchasing and Inventory Management.* Rockville, Md.: Aspen Systems Corporation, 1982.

Schumacher, G.E. "Use of Bioavailability Data by Practitioners: Pitfalls in Interpreting the Data." *American Journal of Hospital Pharmacy* 32 (1975): 839-843.

Trudeau, T., ed. *Topics in Hospital Pharmacy Management* 1, no. 2, 1981.

Chapter 7

Drug Distribution

7

Regardless of whether traditional or unit dose drug dispensing is in effect in an institution, the outcome must be the same: the correct drug and dosage form must be dispensed to the correct patient at the correct time. Because the unit dose dispensing system has been recognized as the "state of the art" in health care in the United States, the scope of this chapter will be limited to this system.[1,2] With some modifications, the QA standards could be adapted for use in other dispensing systems.

In 1974, Beste and DeLeon's article in *Hospitals* defined pharmacy's responsibility in the provision of high-quality health care as the responsibility "related to the medication control process."[3] The authors advise cooperation between nursing service and pharmacy to establish standards for the entire medication process. These policies and procedures should be in both the nursing service and pharmacy manuals. Moreover, yearly review should be conducted with documentation and revision as needed. These policies form the foundation for all medication transactions and are the basis of the QA standards for drug distribution.

The fact that the pharmacy department is responsible for all medications in every department in the hospital is another basic principle. To ensure uniform quality and low cost of all drugs, the pharmacy must control both the purchasing and the distributing functions. The following statement is an example of a standard adopted to enforce this principle: "No drug samples shall be administered to patients in the hospital." This standard usually prevents unauthorized medication use by professional staff or hospitalized patients.

As hospital pharmacy practice evolves toward more patient interaction, the routine distributive functions (e.g., unit dose cart filling) are being carried out under the supervision of a pharmacist by technical support personnel. Since the development of sophisticated clinical pharmacy services depends upon the smooth operation of distributive medication tasks, safeguards and check systems must be an integral part of the dispensing system. The concept of pharmacy-based medication administration teams takes this system one step farther. With these teams, pharmacy controls the drugs from purchase until the ultimate administration to the patients. Therefore, quality assurance is inherent in the medication process and will produce the desired patient outcome and patient safety.

THE PHARMACY PATIENT PROFILE

The pharmacy patient profile is the key document in the unit dose system. The profile provides a complete medication history during the entire hospital stay. It may also be designed as a charging document, providing a record of medication charges to the patient. There are many ways to construct medication profiles, depending upon hospital policies. Listed below are some areas of the profile that can be monitored for accuracy, as part of the QA process:

- patient name and identification number
- patient age and sex
- patient weight
- allergy information
- stop and start dates for medications
- drugs given in other departments (e.g., surgery, recovery, radiology)
- indication of discontinued medications
- indication that all medications are stopped when patient is taken to surgery
- enforcement of stop-order policy for specified drugs
- patient discharge date entered on profile
- verification by pharmacist of orders transcribed by technician
- special designation of controlled substances if required by state law
- correct charging of all medications
- verification by comparison with nursing records that all doses were given.

DRUG ALLERGIES AND DRUG INTERACTION SCREENING

Two specialized items of information should be carefully checked by the pharmacist before any new medication orders are filled. These are drug allergies and potential drug interactions. If drug allergy information on all patients is not being transmitted from nursing personnel to pharmacy, the pharmacist may be able to develop a service that takes patients' medication histories. This situation is a problem that may require a multidisciplinary approach toward finding a solution. It is certainly an opportunity for quality assurance, in which a problem that has been identified may be corrected and documented. Regardless of the approach, the allergy information is required on the nursing and pharmacy medication profiles. This information must be checked before a medication is dispensed and, again, before it is administered.

Drug interaction screening must also be conducted prior to the dispensing of a new medication order. One structural assessment related to this function is to have current references in the dispensing area to facilitate the screening process. A method of documenting communication with physicians should be devised. Documentation prevents repeat calls by other pharmacists for the same interaction. Should any adverse effects develop, the procedure also records the pharmacist's actions to alert the physician. As an assessment technique, patient profiles can be reviewed at a specified interval (e.g., monthly) to look for potential interactions. If any are detected, the communications and documentation should be examined. In the event that a potential interaction, which was not recognized during the patient's therapy, is discovered during the assessment, in-service training can be conducted on the drugs involved. Reaudits can help determine the effectiveness of the screening program and the in-service training.

PROCEDURAL CHECKS

The dispensing procedures lend themselves to process assessment. Using the policy and procedure written for unit dose dispensing, a checklist of safety steps can be designed to ensure accuracy of all doses. Examples of this method of measurement can be found in the *Model Quality Assurance Program for Hospital Pharmacies,* published by the American Society of Hospital Pharmacists,[4] and in an article by Hoffman and associates, published in *Hospital Pharmacy* in July 1980.[5]

If the pharmacy has previously established guidelines for the percent of drugs that must be dispensed in unit dose form, another assessment technique to be considered involves randomly counting the total number of doses dispensed in a set of patient cubicles and determining the percentage of doses in unit dose form. If the result is below the established minimum, a review of the packaging operations is in order.

The Joint Commission on Accreditation of Hospitals (JCAH) specifies that drugs available to nursing service to fill new orders when the pharmacy is closed must be in unit dose form.[6] A regularly scheduled review of these medications should also be conducted. They should be checked for expired drugs, correct and complete labeling, and integrity of each package. The inspection should be documented as usual.

The daily comparison of pharmacy and nursing medication profiles is the heart of the unit dose concept. Since third-party payors use the nursing records to verify medication administration, they may disallow charges on the patient's bill if the pharmacy and nursing records are not in perfect agreement. One of the methods of preventing discrepancies is to reconcile the final nursing medication profile with the pharmacy records at patient discharge. Final billing will then be accurate and complete, reducing the need for credits or late charges.

One method of checking on the accuracy of dispensing, administering, and charting medications was described by Katz.[7] Over a 30- to 60-day period, all medical and surgical patients' unadministered doses returned to the pharmacy were noted. Examination of the reasons for return of the medications led to the discovery of several problems. These reasons were categorized and analyzed so that appropriate corrective actions could be implemented. The study reported by Katz showed that an average of 4.4 to 5.2 percent of medications dispensed was not administered. Some of the reasons for the return of the drug were justified; others were symptoms of problems in the system itself. As Katz points out, "it is not enough to design, develop and implement a unit dose system and then expect that the medications dispensed will be administered as ordered."[8] Unadministered doses should be checked daily and the reasons for each determined if the system is to be completely effective.

Another important aspect to check is the correctness of the administered dose versus the prescribed dose. If the prescribed dose varies in any way from the amount commercially available (e.g., one-half tablet or two capsules), there is a potential for administration of an incorrect dose. Routine checks of this nature, coupled with in-service training and careful labeling, can reduce drug errors dramatically. This is one area in which QA activities have a direct effect upon patient care and patient safety.

INCIDENTS, ADVERSE REACTIONS, AND COMPLAINTS

A periodic review of incident reports pertaining to medication activities can be very educational. It can point out weaknesses in staffing patterns, training, policies, and performance. Appropriate corrective action should address the specific cause of the problem. Reassessment may show an ongoing need for reminders, such as medication classes, newsletters, or other teaching aids.

If there are complaints from patients, nursing, or medical staff, they should be investigated, not only to determine cause but also to detect potential symptoms of a larger problem. For example, if patients are late receiving their 9:00 A.M. medications every day, the cause must be determined. Are medication carts being exchanged during the time that medications are supposed to be administered? Are patients scheduled for tests away from the nursing unit at 9:00 A.M.? Are nurses attending in-service training at 9:00 A.M.? Once the cause is found, it can be determined whether it is part of a larger problem or whether a simple solution is possible.

Errors, incident reports, and adverse reactions are among the topics that should be discussed at pharmacy and therapeutics committee meetings. It is important to keep these incidents in perspective. The error rate should be compared with the total number of doses dispensed in a given time period. Errors should be used as a source of learning experience, not as an excuse to point an accusing finger at other professionals.

Adverse drug reactions should be documented in the patient's chart and brought to the pharmacist's and physician's attention. It may be necessary to contact the product manufacturer or the Food and Drug Administration if the adverse effect is thought to be due to a product defect. Analysis of such incidents might lead to a review of the sources of specific products, if the frequency or severity of reactions warrants it.

COMMUNICATIONS

There are many opportunities for the pharmacist to communicate with other professionals and patients to impart specialized information. Some of these are mandated (e.g., by Medicare and JCAH regulations).[9,10] The quality of these communications helps to determine how other professionals perceive the pharmacist's competence. Measuring the effectiveness and frequency of these presentations should be part of the QA program. Examples of types of communication methods are given below:

- newsletters for medical, nursing, and pharmacy staff
- in-service programs
- continuing education programs
- patient counseling
- orientation to pharmacy for new pharmacy and nursing personnel
- medication history
- patient rounds with medical staff
- attendance at infection control, pharmacy and therapeutics, head nurse, patient care, safety, and utilization review committee meetings
- attendance at medical staff meetings, pathological conferences, QA committee meetings
- discussions with physicians and nurses regarding specific therapy situations
- presentation of programs to the community.

Documentation of these information exchanges can be used for the following purposes:

- to show inspectors and meet regulatory requirements for these activities
- to justify pharmacy services and personnel
- to measure abilities and knowledge of pharmacists
- to teach procedures and drug-related information
- to share new information with others
- to demonstrate willingness of pharmacists to learn and to teach
- to improve the level of care provided to the patient.

CONTROLLED SUBSTANCES

In Chapters 2 and 6, the regulations and record-keeping requirements for controlled drugs are discussed. Since these drugs are so carefully regulated, they are natural components of the drug distribution QA functions.

One area to monitor involves drugs dispensed on a proof-of-use sheet for nurses to sign. Periodic checks on sheets still on the nursing unit can reveal the need to revise stock levels and delete slow-moving items. Following an audit trail of doses from purchasing, through dispensing, to charting can be an excellent method of auditing each part of the dispensing process.

Another area of control, which may be difficult to enforce, involves those controlled substances on floor stock that are subject to the stop order policy (e.g., narcotics and hypnotics). Despite the notification of nursing and medical staff that the order must be renewed before the patient can receive more, the nurse may continue to administer the drug as needed from the floor stock supply. This is another multidisciplinary problem requiring various professionals working together to find a solution.

Another review that can be very enlightening is a check on controlled drugs returned in the patient's medication cubicle after the patient's dismissal from the hospital. Are all unadministered doses present? Have some been sent home with the patient or not labeled by the pharmacy with directions for use? Are controlled drugs dispensed in the cubicle always returned to the pharmacy?

Since the most traditional functions conducted by pharmacists involve dispensing, this is often the first area for development of QA standards. The most familiar aspect of services rendered is the best place to begin. Sharing the development of the QA standards for dispensing allows the staff to participate and accept the guidelines for everyone's activities. Involvement of nursing personnel ensures that all aspects of the system are included. Understanding the rules helps all team members to strive for mutually desired goals.

NOTES

1. Michael H. Stolar, "National Survey of Hospital Pharmacy Services—1978," *American Journal of Hospital Pharmacy* 36 (1979): 316-324.

2. "ASHP Statement on Unit Dose Drug Distribution," *American Journal of Hospital Pharmacy* 38, no. 8 (1981): 1214.

3. Donald F. Beste, Jr. and Richard F. DeLeon, "Medication Process: Who's Responsible?" *Hospitals* 48 (March 1, 1974): 97-100.

4. *Model Quality Assurance Program for Hospital Pharmacies* (Washington, D.C.: American Society of Hospital Pharmacists, 1978), pp. 9-14.

5. Richard P. Hoffman et al., "Development of a Multi-hospital Pharmacy Quality Assurance Program," *Hospital Pharmacy* 15 (1980): 365-380.

6. *Accreditation Manual for Hospitals* (Chicago: Joint Commission on Accreditation of Hospitals, 1980), pp. 137-145.

7. Elaine Katz, "Unadministered Medications in a Unit Dose System," *Quality Review Bulletin* special edition (Summer 1981), pp. 44-48.

8. Ibid., p. 48.

9. Ibid.

10. "Conditions for Participation," Medicare Regulations (Washington, D.C.: Department of Health, Education and Welfare, 1969), publication no. 19,821, Reg. Sec. 405.1027.

SUGGESTED READINGS

Model QA Program for Hospital Pharmacies. Washington, D.C.: American Society of Hospital Pharmacists, 1978.

Sourcebook on Unit Dose Drug Distribution Systems. Washington, D.C.: American Society of Hospital Pharmacists, 1978.

White, Sara J., and Godwin, Harold N. "A Unit Dose Quality Assurance Program." *Hospital Pharmacy* 12 (1977): 90-96.

Chapter 8

Preparation of Sterile Products

8

The need for quality assurance has probably been demonstrated most dramatically in the field of intravenous admixtures. In Chapter 1, several examples were cited showing the potential for harm that exists when there are no controls on admixture techniques. This lack of controls was summarized by Zellmer in an editorial published in the May 1978 issue of the *American Journal of Hospital Pharmacy*.[1] Zellmer called for a formal QA program to include checks on accuracy, sterility techniques, and the training of employees who prepare admixtures.

In an article in the same issue entitled, "Evaluation of Compounding Accuracy and Aseptic Techniques for Intravenous Admixtures," Sanders and associates demonstrated the urgent need for monitoring admixture techniques.[2] In Stage I of the experiment, both pharmacists and technicians were observed while compounding admixtures; every participant committed at least one error: the pharmacists showed an error rate of 34.4 percent, while technicians had a 56.6 percent error rate.

The process was repeated in Stage II, with personnel informed that they were being observed and evaluated. The results for Stage II were error rates of 36.6 percent for pharmacists and 43.3 percent for technicians. None of the 21 participants in both stages of the study was error free; furthermore, not one quantitative analysis of admixture solutions yielded a drug content in exact agreement with the labeled amount of that ingredient! While there are many factors that may cause these variations, the fact that they exist strengthens the case for a QA program.

Decreased federal spending for health care programs has defunded one of the external source of controls (i.e., the National Coordinating Committee on Large Volume Parenterals [NCCLVP]). This is one more vital reason for internal controls.

When designing the QA program for sterile products, it is essential to ensure that all the elements of the program be included. Stolar's article in the *American*

Journal of Hospital Pharmacy in May 1979 outlined five general areas to be monitored in the pharmacy's QA plan:[3]

1. appropriateness of the admixture order
2. product sterility
3. freedom from particulate contamination
4. correct ingredients and amounts in solutions
5. proper labeling, storage, and distribution.

The reader is referred to this article for suggestions of items to consider in each of these categories. Some other topics that might be evaluated for inclusion in the QA plan are also presented in this chapter.

SCREENING NEW INTRAVENOUS SOLUTION ORDERS

Some of the pharmacist's more important tasks in preparing admixtures occur *before* the technical activities are carried out. For example, the physician's order must be reviewed in detail and screened for any or all of the following items:

- appropriateness of the order for the patient
- duplications of therapy (e.g., patient taking the same drug orally)
- drug allergies
- special conditions (e.g., diabetes or low sodium intake) that limit solutions to be administered
- potential drug interactions
- method of administration (e.g., peripheral versus central administration)
- incompatibilities of prescribed drugs or drugs and solution
- total fluid intake prescribed.

The discussion in Chapter 7 relating to screening patients' medication orders in the drug distribution system is also applicable to the processes used for admixtures. To assist the pharmacist, incompatibility guides and other references should be present in the admixture area. A retrospective review of patient profiles and labels on solution containers can be useful for determining the effectiveness of screening activities. Sample QA standards and their respective assessment methodologies for these professional activities are shown in Exhibit 8-1.

Exhibit 8-1 Sterile Preparations QA Standards for Professional Activities

STANDARD	QUESTION	YES/NO	METHODOLOGY
1. There are no errors in the preparation and in the dispensing of sterile preparations.	How many errors have been reported in the preparation and/or dispensing of sterile preparations?		Record errors reported over a 14-day period.
2. The laminar flow hood will be inspected and certified at least every 12 months.	What was date of last inspection & certification?		
3. There are no known allergies to drugs being administered.	Is there a mechanism for screening medication allergies of specific drug entities? Describe. How many doses of medication were dispensed to patients known to be allergic to the drug dispensed? How many doses of medication were administered to patients known to be allergic to the drug administered?		Record number of doses dispensed and number of doses administered to known allergic patients over a 14-day period.
4. There are no undetected clinically significant physical, chemical or therapeutic incompatibilities of sterile preparations.	Is there a mechanism for screening for potential physical, chemical or therapeutic incompatibilities or interactions prior to dispensing? Describe. How many clinically significant interactions were detected prior to dispensing?		Document incompatibilities detected for a 14-day period.

Source: HPI Hospital Pharmacies, Inc., Sterile Preparations Assessment Report, © 1980. Reprinted with permission.

INFECTION CONTROL

The subject of infection control in intravenous admixture preparation has been covered in great detail in the literature.[4,5] The program in the pharmacy begins with the acceptance and implementation of policies and procedures for personnel preparing admixtures. These include aspects such as:

- handwashing
- prevention of administration or admixture preparation by employees having an infection
- culturing admixtures and laminar flow hood surfaces
- inspection of solution containers for cracks or signs of contamination.

Monitoring adherence to these policies is an integral part of the QA program. For guidelines relating to sterility testing of admixtures, the reader is referred to the suggested readings at the end of the chapter. A complete review of the guidelines established by the NCCLVP is advisable to ensure that every facet of admixture procedures is included in the QA plan.[6]

Another mechanism involves checking to see whether any patient developing a nosocomial infection had received intravenous therapy. Correlation of this data can detect problems and suggest causes. A procedure must be established to outline methods for the pharmacy and infection control personnel to use for following up a suspected admixture-related infection. Sample QA standards pertaining to infection control are shown in Exhibit 8-2.

Both large and small volume parenterals must be included whenever inventory is inspected for expired products. These products are also included when reporting defects to the Food and Drug Administration (FDA). In addition, a policy must be established for the length of use of multidose injectable vials once they have been opened.

TRAINING OF PERSONNEL AND RELATED ELEMENTS

Standard III of the Joint Commission on Accreditation of Hospitals (JCAH) standards for pharmaceutical services specifies the need for formal training of those personnel preparing admixtures.[7] Individuals responsible for preparing admixtures need training in two types of techniques: (1) compounding accuracy and (2) aseptic manipulations. Not only do pharmacy personnel need this instruction, but any nurse who prepares admixtures when the pharmacy is closed should also receive this training. Both initial orientation and subsequent in-service education are mentioned in the JCAH standard. Documentation of orientation, in-

Exhibit 8-2 Sterile Preparations QA Standards for Infection Control

STANDARD	QUESTION	YES/NO
1. All sterile preparations <u>are</u> sterile.	Do you test for sterility of finished products? Describe process of sterility testing. How many positive cultures have been reported in last 90 days?	
2. The laminar flow hood is cleaned at least once per shift and documented.	Is the hood cleaned at the beginning of each shift?	
3. The laminar flow hood will be cultured routinely and documented.	What type of microbiological monitoring is required by the Infection Control Committee? Describe.	
4. The pre-filter will be changed or cleaned not less than monthly (more often if necessary) with documentation.	How often is the pre-filter changed?	

Source: HPI Hospital Pharmacies, Inc., Sterile Preparations Assessment Report, © 1980. Reprinted with permission.

service education, annual review, and evaluation of admixture and nursing personnel can be built into the QA plan.

The manufacturers of intravenous fluids can be helpful in providing training seminars and educational materials to assist in orientation of personnel.[8] These resources can be obtained by contacting local representatives of the solution manufacturers or by sending requests addressed to their respective medical education departments.

Labeling of intravenous admixture containers by pharmacy personnel should include specific elements, as suggested by the American Society of Hospital Pharmacists (ASHP).[9] Random checks of actual labels, compared with the ASHP requirements, will provide an ongoing validation of accuracy. A sample of a QA standard written to monitor labeling compliance is illustrated in Exhibit 8-3.

The problem of particulate matter in admixtures cannot be overlooked.[10,11] Hospital policy should include delineation of admixtures that require administra-

Exhibit 8-3 Sterile Preparations QA Standards for Labeling Intravenous Admixtures

STANDARD	QUESTION	YES/NO
1. Labeling information:	What information is routinely put on labels for all IV admixtures leaving the pharmacy?	
1.1 All IV admixtures leaving the pharmacy have the following labeled information:		
1.1.1 Patient and room number	Patient and room number ______	
1.1.2 Name of drug as ordered (on label or communication form to nursing for insertion on their medication profile).	Name of drug as ordered (on label or communication form to nursing for insertion on nursing medication profile).	
1.1.3 Strength, concentration or volume	Strength or concentration or volume ______	
1.1.4 Expiration date or date of preparation	Expiration date or date of preparation with published expiration policy.	
1.1.5 Initials of verifying pharmacist.	Initials of verifying pharmacist ______	
1.1.6 Auxiliary labels (when necessary)	Auxiliary labels (when necessary)______	
1.1.7 Solution name	Solution name ______	

Source: HPI Hospital Pharmacies, Inc., Sterile Preparations Assessment Report, © 1980. Reprinted with permission.

tion using a 0.45- or 0.22-micron filter. Pharmacy policy should also dictate which drugs require preparation using a filter (e.g., any drug from a glass ampule). Adherence to these policies can also be verified by the QA methodology.

The use of infusion devices, such as pumps and controllers, must also be established by hospital policy. Intensive training of all who use or maintain the equipment should be followed by monitoring to ensure correct usage. Standards can also be established for care and maintenance of the infusion devices. Examples of the type of standards that apply to maintenance of infusion devices are shown in Exhibit 8-4.

Exhibit 8-4 Sample QA Standards for Maintenance of Infusion Devices

STANDARD	QUESTION	YES	NO	N/A
1. There is documentation of in-service education on all types of infusion devices for nursing and pharmacy staff.	Do you have documentation of in-service education to: Nursing staff? Pharmacy Staff?			
2. There shall be routine mechanical checks of each device, with documentation of the procedures.	Are there routine mechanical checks of devices? How often? Is there documentation of these checks?			
3. There is documentation of any device malfunction, with corrective action taken.	Is documentation of device malfunction maintained? Is corrective action documented?			
4. There is documentation of device usage.	How is device usage documented? Describe.			
5. All infusion devices shall receive at least quarterly electrical inspection, to include: • leakage of current • verification of integrity of power cords and strain relief devices. Documentation of these procedures is to be kept in the pharmacy (e.g., sticker on equipment or written record).	Do all infusion devices receive at least quarterly electrical inspections? How is this procedure documented?			
6. There are written policies and procedures for the following: 6.1 Device set-up and calibration. 6.2 Periodic mechanical checks.	Do you have approved policies and procedures for each topic 6.1 through 6.8?			

Exhibit 8-4 continued

6.3 In-service education on use of devices.				
6.4 Priority of use.				
6.5 Trouble-shooting for possible malfunction.				
6.6 Maintenance and repair of devices.				
6.7 Distribution of devices and location.				
6.8 Cleaning and decontamination of devices.				

Source: HPI Hospital Pharmacies, Inc., Sterile Preparations Assessment Report, © 1981. Reprinted with permission.

There has been a great deal of concern expressed in the literature about the safety of the personnel who handle chemotherapeutic agents.[12,13] The training of those individuals preparing these products must certainly include safety measures for handling toxic substances. It is in the best interest of the individual to comply with these procedures. A good risk management program will include safe methods of handling such agents.

INTERACTION WITH OTHER PROFESSIONALS

Because intravenous therapy, like other facets of patient care, involves various health care professionals, it is prudent to consider the quality of the interactions of pharmacy personnel with these individuals. The multidisciplinary relationships of health care professionals are evident from the very beginning of the planning, through implementation, to the day-to-day functions of patient care.

Other professionals involved in the care of a patient receiving IV therapy may include medical staff, nursing, laboratory, infection control, business office, radiology, central service, surgery, recovery room, dietary, and intravenous therapy team members, as well as those in the pharmacy. Standards can be developed to measure accuracy and timeliness of services provided by these departments or by the pharmacy to these departments. A more detailed discussion of this subject is provided in Chapter 11. A few examples are listed in Table 8-1.

Table 8-1 Services Provided to Patients Receiving Intravenous Therapy

DEPARTMENT	SERVICE
Infection Control	Culture and sensitivity reports Incidence of nosocomial infection Resistance and susceptibility of organisms to antibiotics
Laboratory	Electrolyte and other test results Culture reports of admixtures, pharmacy equipment, etc. Culture and sensitivity reports Drug levels
Nursing Service	IV flow charts Tubing and dressing changes Administration of blood or components Initiation and discontinuation of IV therapy Changes in physician orders Assessment of patient's status Administration of IV "push" drugs Prevention of infiltration, occlusion, etc. Use of infusion devices
Medical Staff	Initiation and discontinuation of IV therapy Appropriate fluid and additive dose and route of administration Special precautions, e.g., fluid restriction Assessment of nutritional and fluid balance status
Radiology	Administration of contrast media Assurance of correct catheter placement

Table 8-1 continued

DEPARTMENT	SERVICE
Pharmacy	Review of physician orders
	Preparation of admixtures
	Charging for admixture services and elements
	Assessment of benefits and hazards of therapy
	Consultation with professionals and patients
	Assurance of sterility
	Provision of training

The need for QA standards as a guide for the IV therapist has long been established in the literature.[14-16] Whether the IV team reports to pharmacy, nursing, or any other department, it is appropriate for the pharmacist to play an active role in developing QA standards for intravenous therapy.

A model QA program for IV therapists was devised at Spartanburg General Hospital in Spartanburg, South Carolina. Comparison of daily IV-related activities for intravenous therapy team members and for nonteam nurses showed a significantly higher level of performance and knowledge for the IV team members. However, the author points out that "you do not know if you have sacrificed quality for efficiency unless you have a quality assurance program."[17] The reader is referred to this article for examples of structure, process, and outcome standards for determining the quality of IV therapy services.

TOTAL PARENTERAL NUTRITION AND OTHER SPECIALIZED SERVICES

Standards for assessment of the quality of clinical pharmacy services are among the newest areas to be developed. This subject is discussed in greater detail in Chapter 12.

The area of special services provides opportunities for the pharmacist to consult with nursing and medical staff on protocols, potential problems, and procedures. Documentation of these activities can produce data for assessment of the quality of clinical services.

Parenteral nutrition, for example, provides a wealth of parameters to monitor, both for nursing and pharmacy. Sample criteria for monitoring of total parenteral nutrition are given in Table 8-2.

Table 8-2 Sample Criteria for Monitoring Parenteral Nutrition

CRITERIA	IDEAL COMPLIANCE	EXCEPTIONS	DATA SOURCE
1. Formalized nutritional assessment is performed prior to therapy and/or at least every three weeks during therapy.	100%	None	Progress notes, physician's order sheet, flow sheet
2. Chest X-ray shows tip of catheter to be within superior venacava, prior to initiation of solution administration.	100%	None	Progress notes, radiology reports
3. Daily weight intake and output are measured and recorded.	100%	None	Order sheet, flow sheet, nursing notes
4. Catheter dressing is changed at least three times per week, according to hospital policy.	100%	None	Order sheet, nursing notes, progress notes
5. Incidence of complications:			
5.1 Hypoglycemia (blood sugar less than 80mg%)	0%	None	Nursing MAR, lab reports, flow sheet, progress notes
5.2 Hyperglycemia (blood sugar greater than 200mg%)	0%	None	Nursing MAR, lab reports, flow sheet, progress notes
5.3 Febrile reaction (temperature greater than 101° during at least two readings within 24 hours)	0%	None	Progress notes, temperature record

Source: HPI Quality Assurance Program, Audit Criteria for Parenteral Nutrition (Central), © 1981. Reprinted with permission.

Some of the other special services that can be included in an admixture program (and, therefore, in the QA program) include:

- use of infusion devices
- chemotherapy
- administration of medications via heparin lock
- investigational drug protocols

- administration of blood components
- use of filters
- special restrictions (e.g., low sodium intake).

In each case, standards can be developed to measure effectiveness of the pharmacist's intervention in the patient's intravenous therapy.

RECORD-KEEPING REQUIREMENTS

As in any other sphere of pharmacy practice, intravenous admixture services require certain documentation activities. A list of some of the areas that require record keeping is given below. Examples of a few QA standards covering this area are illustrated in Exhibit 8-5.

- lot number of solutions and additives for each patient
- patient profile entries of intravenous therapy
- records of laminar flow hood cleaning and annual maintenance
- refrigerator temperature record
- documentation of training and evaluation of those preparing admixtures
- in-service programs
- hood and admixture culture records.

The fact that intravenous drugs are, by definition, administered directly into the bloodstream, demonstrates the value of the safeguards to the patient provided by the QA standards covering this domain. The precept "first do no harm" must be the guiding principle for everyone involved in patient care.

Exhibit 8-5 Sterile Preparations QA Standards for Record Keeping

STANDARD	QUESTION	YES/NO
1. There is a way of determining the manufacturer, manufacturer's lot number and preparer of ingredients and vehicles for each IV admixture.	Do you record manufacturer, manufacturer's lot number and preparer for ingredients and vehicles for IV admixtures? Describe procedure briefly.	
2. All medication error incident reports are reviewed by pharmacy.	Are you made aware of all medication errors reported? Do you take appropriate action? Describe.	
3. There shall be routine mechanical checks of each infusion device, with documentation of the procedures.	Are there routine mechanical checks of devices? How often? Is there documentation of of these checks?	
4. There is documentation of infusion device usage.	How is infusion device usage documented?	
5. There is documentation of any infusion malfunction with corrective action taken.	Is documentation of device malfunction and corrective action maintained?	
6. There is documentation of in-service education on all types of infusion devices for nursing and pharmacy staff.	Do you have documentation of in-service education for: • Nursing staff • Pharmacy staff	

Source: HPI Hospital Pharmacies, Inc., Sterile Preparations Reassessment Report, © 1981. Reprinted with permission.

NOTES

1. William Zellmer, "Quality Control in Admixture Services," *American Journal of Hospital Pharmacy* 35 (1978): 527-528.

2. Lonnie H. Sanders et al., "Evaluation of Compounding Accuracy and Aseptic Techniques for Intravenous Admixtures," *American Journal of Hospital Pharmacy* 35 (1978): 531-536.

3. Michael H. Stolar, "Assuring the Quality of Intravenous Admixtures Programs," *American Journal of Hospital Pharmacy* 36 (1979): 605-608.

4. Donald A. Goldman et al., "Guidelines for Infection Control in Intravenous Therapy," *Annals of Internal Medicine* 79, no. 6 (1973): 848-850.

5. Salvatore J. Turco, "Quality Assurance in IV Admixture Programs," *Hospital Pharmacy* 14 (1979): 307-313.

6. National Coordinating Committee on Large Volume Parenterals, "Recommended Guidelines for Quality Assurance in Hospital Centralized Intravenous Admixture Services," *American Journal of Hospital Pharmacy* 37 (1980): 645.

7. *Accreditation Manual for Hospitals* (Chicago: Joint Commission on Accreditation of Hospitals, 1980), pp. 132-145.

8. Max Hunt, *Training Manual for Central Intravenous Admixture Personnel* (Morton Grove, Ill.: Travenol Laboratories, 1972).

9. "Recommendations for the Labeling of Large Volume Parenterals," *American Journal of Hospital Pharmacy* 35 (1978): 49.

10. Robert Rapp, B. Bivins, and P. DeLuca, "Filtration and IV Therapy," *IV Therapy and Clinical Nutrition* 7, no. 4 (1980): 36-46.

11. "Problems and Benefits of In-Line Filtration," National Coordinating Committee on Large Volume Parenterals, publication no. 79-01, November 30, 1979.

12. R.S. Knowles and J.E. Verdon, "Handling of Injectable Antineoplastic Agents," *British Medical Journal* 281 (1980): 589-591.

13. Salvatore J. Turco, "Cancer Chemotherapeutic Agents: Handling and Disposal," *Infusion*, February 1981, p. 6.

14. N.J. Magel, "Quality Assurance and IV Therapy," *American Journal of Intravenous Therapy and Clinical Nutrition* 8, no. 1 (1981): 11-23.

15. "The Standards of Practice of the American Association of Intravenous Therapy," *American Journal of Intravenous Therapy and Clinical Nutrition* 6, no. 5 (1979): 27-33.

16. National Intravenous Therapy Association, Inc., "Standards of Practice," *NITA, Journal of National Intravenous Therapy Association* 3, no. 4 (1980): 133-138.

17. Cheryl Gardner, "Quality Assurance Control in IV Therapy," *NITA, Journal of National Intravenous Therapy Association* 4, no. 1 (1981): 28-36.

SUGGESTED READINGS

Canter, L.P. "Cost Justifying the Implementation of IV Teams." *NITA, Journal of National Intravenous Therapy Association* 3, no. 6 (1980): 217-232.

Gormecan, Annette. "Audit of Dietary Care Shows Better Documentation Needed." *Hospitals* 44, no. 6 (March 16, 1981): 107-110.

Hansten, Philip D. *Drug Interactions*, 4th ed. Philadelphia: Lea & Febiger, 1979.

Infection Control in the Hospital. Chicago: American Hospital Association, 1979, pp. 58-61 and 166-168.

James, John D., et al. *A Guide to Drug Interactions.* New York: McGraw Hill Book Company, 1978.

Jarocha, Henry. "Microbiological Quality Control in a Hospital Pharmacy." *Hospital Pharmacy* 12 (1977): 575-581.

Kaminski, Mitchell V., Jr., and Stolar, Michael H. "Parenteral Hyperalimentation—A Quality of Care Survey and Review. *American Journal of Hospital Pharmacy* 31 (1974): 228-235.

Kilarski, David J., et al. "Use Review of Intravenous Infusion Devices." *American Journal of Hospital Pharmacy* 38 (1981): 1517-1518.

King, James C. *Guide to Parenteral Admixtures.* St. Louis: Cutter Laboratories, 1978.

Martin, Eric W. *Hazards of Medication,* 2nd ed. Philadelphia: J.B. Lippincott, 1978.

Mayhall, C.G., et al. "Evaluation of a Device for Monitoring Sterility of Injectable Fluids." *American Journal of Hospital Pharmacy* 38 (1981): 1148-1150.

National Coordinating Committee on Large Volume Parenterals. "Recommended Procedures for In-Use Testing of Large Volume Parenterals Suspected of Contamination or of Producing a Reaction in a Patient." *American Journal of Hospital Pharmacy* 35 (1978): 678-682.

Trissel, L.A. *Pocket Guide to Injectable Drugs.* Washington, D.C.: American Society of Hospital Pharmacists, 1981.

Wilson, Jacqueline A. "Infection Control in Intravenous Therapy." *Heart and Lung* 4, no. 3 (1976): 430-436.

Chapter 9

Policy and Procedure Manual

9

REQUIREMENTS FOR THE MANUAL

The policy and procedure manual can be one of the most dynamic and vital pieces of documentation in any department of the hospital. Unfortunately, its only reason for existence in many departments is the certainty that it will be examined by an inspector from one of the regulatory agencies that audit health care facilities.

While it is true that a policy and procedure manual for the pharmacy department is required in several guidelines, it has definite intrinsic value as a reference for department personnel. The "Minimum Standards for Pharmacies in Institutions," approved by the American Society of Hospital Pharmacists (ASHP) in 1977, specifies the need for an operational manual to govern all pharmacy functions.[1] This manual is to be continually revised, and all department personnel should be familiar with its contents. It should also specify lines of authority and areas of responsibility for the department.[2]

The American Hospital Association (AHA) stated the purposes of the policy and procedure manual in 1970.[3] The manual is designed to "promote safe and consistent performance of particular acts or functions by all personnel within the department."[4] Further, it should "acquaint other hospital departments with pharmacy policies and procedures, thereby reducing confusion and possible interdepartmental friction."[5] Hassan recommends developing the pharmacy's manual to include four main sections:[6]

1. organization of the hospital and the pharmacy
2. equipment and physical plant
3. personnel policies
4. department services and activities

- administrative (e.g., hours of operation records, controls, and reports)
- professional (e.g., services provided, drug information, dispensing, and purchasing).

Regardless of the organization of the manual, the elements listed above should be included. Careful review of the Joint Commission on Accreditation of Hospitals (JCAH) standards for pharmaceutical services will enable the pharmacist to establish a list of subjects to include in the manual.[7] As new services are developed, or existing ones are modified, the manual should be revised accordingly.

REVIEW, REVISION, AND ANNUAL APPROVAL

The pharmacy's policy and procedure manual is never complete. Since the practice of hospital pharmacy is a dynamic discipline, the manual must always be in a state of revision, in order to keep it current and reflecting actual practice. It is advisable, therefore, to select a format that facilitates revision, such as a loose-leaf binder. The numbering of pages should permit insertion and deletion of pages without affecting the organization of the manual.[8]

A policy should be established to ensure that individuals or departments that require a copy of the manual receive one, and the policy should include a mechanism to keep the manual current. The latter should define those who can initiate changes, how they are accomplished, who reviews and approves them, and listings of provisions made for storage of deleted materials. A mechanism in the QA plan of the department should ensure that every copy of the manual has new pages inserted and obsolete pages removed.[9]

The entire manual should be reviewed and approved annually by the Pharmacy and Therapeutics Committee.[10] The title page of the manual is usually used to display this approval, indicated by the signature of the Director of Pharmacy, Administrator, Chairman of the Pharmacy and Therapeutics Committee, Chief of Medical Staff, and any others deemed appropriate in the by-laws of the hospital.

In addition, it should be possible to determine when any particular policy was written, approved, reviewed, or revised. Various methods can be used to provide this documentation, as shown in Exhibits 9-1 through 9-3. Each of the methods has its advantages and disadvantages. Writing approval and revision dates on the page itself provides an easy method for locating this information. On the other hand, retyping policies will be required more frequently, since this method tends to detract from the appearance.

The pages showing when a policy was approved, reviewed, or revised are quite efficient and easy to use. All this information is collected in one section of the manual, enabling the pharmacist to determine which policies require attention.

Exhibit 9-1 Policy and Procedure Documentation Device

Policy number......

Approval Date__________

Review Date __________

Revision Date__________

Exhibit 9-2 Policy and Procedure Revision Record

	JAN	FEB	MAR	APR	MAY	JUNE
Hours of Operation		Reviewed				
Interaction Monitoring					Revised	
Library				Reviewed		

Exhibit 9-3 Policy and Procedure Review and Revision Record

	APPROVED	REVIEWED	REVISED	REVISED	REVISED
5.0 After hours dispensing	1979	1980			1981
6.0 Bedside medications	1978	1979	1980	1981	
7.0 Controlled Substance procedures	1981				
8.0 Emergency drug supplies	1980	1981			
9.0 Errors, medication	1979	1980	1981		

This should be built into the QA plan as part of the annual reassessment mechanism.

The use of a duplicate set of table of contents pages without the page numbers provides an overview of all the policies at once. The current status of each can be seen at a glance. It is also possible to see which are new policies or procedures by reviewing the approval dates. This type of documentation is not only valuable to the pharmacist but also facilitates the inspection of the manual by the Pharmacy and Therapeutics Committee or by a representative of any agency that may audit the department.

ENSURING THAT THE MANUAL IS READY FOR INSPECTION

As part of the QA program for the pharmacy, the policy and procedure manual must be reviewed and approved annually. If a checklist of required elements is prepared and used at specified time intervals, the manual will continue to be current. The elements on the checklist can be assembled from JCAH standards, ASHP guidelines, and hospital bylaws. When an inspection is anticipated, such as during biannual visits of inspectors from the JCAH, the pharmacist can review the checklist and ensure the presence of all required items of documentation. An excerpt from such a checklist is shown in Exhibit 9-4.

Exhibit 9-4 Reassessment Report for Pharmacy Activities

	Developed			Approved			Implemented			Documented		
	YES	NO	N/A	YES	NO	N/A	YES	NO	N/A	YES	NO	N/A
POLICY & PROCEDURE MANUAL												
The following Items Shall Be Included in the Policy and Procedure Manual:												
Abbreviations, Approved												
Accountability of Pharmaceutical Service												
Adverse Drug Reactions												
Administrative Reports												
After Hours Dispensing												
Antibiotic Review												
Antidotes and Poisons												
Audits, Nursing Station and Medication Areas												
Audits, Emergency Drug Supply												
Authorized Area for Outdated or Unusable Drugs												
Automatic Stop Orders												
Cancellation of Orders When Patient Goes to Surgery												
Cleaning and Maintenance												
Code Blue Team Participation												

Source: HPI Hospital Pharmacies, Inc., Reassessment Report for Pharmacy Activities, © 1980. Reprinted with permission.

There is another benefit to be achieved by requiring this biannual review of the manual. Reviewing the manual affords the pharmacist an opportunity to reevaluate each policy and procedure for its appropriateness in light of current practice.

It is very important to read and know the department manual *before* the inspector arrives. Past history has shown that pharmacists are often asked to describe a department procedure, after which the inspector compares the written statement in the manual with the verbal account. This is another reason to keep the manual up to date.

BENEFITS OF A POLICY AND PROCEDURE MANUAL

Smith and Brown examined the hospital pharmacy manual and delineated its value.[11] They stated that the policy and procedure manual is:

- the foundation for departmental administrative and professional activities
- the coordination of the department's resources
- a means to improve communication between pharmacy personnel
- a means to inform employees of what is expected of them, which improves morale and performance levels
- a management tool to measure performance versus written standards
- a method to measure the quality of the services being provided by the pharmacy.

The last two points demonstrate how the manual can be used as an assessment tool in the QA program for the pharmacy.

The *Reference Manual on Hospital Pharmacy* provides a different perspective on the value of the manual.[12] Policy and procedure manuals, and evidence of compliance with them, may be presented in civil court cases as proof that the hospital has taken due precautions to ensure that standards of practice protecting patient safety have been met.

Since the JCAH and the AHA both specify that the pharmacy will have a policy and procedure manual, the pharmacist can use this to further the goals of the department. Intradepartmental and multidisciplinary communications are required to write, approve, and implement new policies. Annual review by the Pharmacy and Therapeutics Committee can be used to renew awareness by medical staff of pharmacy activities and capabilities. By comparing the achievements of the past year with the goals established at the beginning of the year, the accomplishments of the pharmacy can be publicized. Thus, the ever-changing, time-consuming manual can be one of the cornerstones of the pharmacy's QA program.

NOTES

1. "Minimum Standards for Pharmacies in Institutions" (Washington, D.C.: American Society of Hospital Pharmacists, August 1977).

2. Ibid.

3. *Reference Manual on Hospital Pharmacy* (Chicago: American Hospital Association, 1970), pp. 15-16.

4. Ibid.

5. Ibid.

6. William E. Hassan, Jr., *Hospital Pharmacy*, 2nd ed. (Philadelphia: Lea & Febiger, 1967), pp. 137-146.

7. *Accreditation Manual for Hospitals* (Chicago: Joint Commission on Accreditation of Hospitals, 1981), pp. 142-145.

8. Mickey C. Smith and Thomas R. Brown, *Handbook of Institutional Pharmacy Practice* (Baltimore: Williams & Wilkins, 1979), pp. 34-51.

9. Ibid.

10. *Accreditation Manual for Hospitals*, pp. 142-145.

11. Smith and Brown, *Handbook*, pp. 34-51.

12. *Reference Manual on Hospital Pharmacy*, pp. 15-16.

Chapter 10

Management Activities

10

Medicine is the only profession that labors incessantly to destroy the reason for its own existence.

—Lord Bryce

A health care manager in a contemporary hospital has a challenging situation to control. Not only do the technical aspects of the services rendered require the manager's attention, but the personnel and regulatory aspects also demand monitoring. Quality assurance, therefore, can be useful to assess both management functions and clinical or operational activities. This chapter will review specific areas of management that quality assurance can measure. The value of QA as a management tool will be discussed in Chapter 17.

The following fable is presented to demonstrate how quality assurance functions for the manager:

Smokey, the King

Long ago, there lived a king who ruled a small, isolated, rural monarchy. One day he called all his counselors and advisors together. "See here," the king said. "The fire department of our kingdom has had so many fires to fight that they never have time to shine up the engine or to play checkers. We are going to develop a program of fire prevention and quality control in this kingdom!"

The king's edict struck fear in the hearts of the assembled leaders. They ran around in circles, lamenting and wringing their hands. Finally, one counselor stepped forward and suggested that they work together to develop a set of goals and action plans to achieve them. Relieved to have some direction, the other statesmen agreed to meet and to begin to develop the required programs.

Once the strategies were implemented, each leader delegated responsibility for carrying out the activities to subordinates in their respective departments in the kingdom. All went well for a few weeks. Then the king called for a council meeting once again. "Can anyone explain why we have had a sudden rash of fires in the last week?" the king demanded. The advisors looked at each other in astonishment. How could this happen? Hadn't they delegated tasks for fire prevention to responsible subordinates? Charged with the task of finding the cause of the problem, the leaders returned to their departments. To their dismay, they found that when the fire prevention tasks had become part of the daily routine, the workers began carrying them out less frequently. Once it became clear that no one was checking on the performance of the chores, the workers ceased doing them completely.

The council met again and established performance criteria as part of a program of quality assurance. Results of assessments were to be reported to the council and to the king on a scheduled basis. Soon the firemen in the kingdom were able to keep the fire engine polished for its appearances in parades, since the number of fires was greatly diminished (see Figure 10-1).

Figure 10-1 Smokey, the King

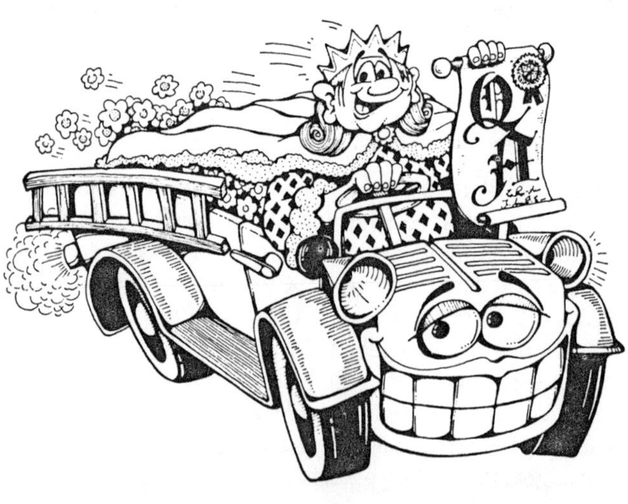

Lessons to be learned from this fable:

1. The problem isn't really solved if it reoccurs.
2. A manager cannot be certain of the quality of the services rendered unless that service is assessed and compared to established standards.
3. Firemen who spend all their time fighting fires never get to ride in the parade.

The story points out that managers, whether in a hospital or a legendary kingdom, have certain responsibilities that cannot be abdicated. The manager, although not responsible for actually performing technical work, nevertheless maintains the accountability for the completion of assigned tasks.

The functions of a manager in any business, industry, or profession have certain components in common. They are planning, leading, organizing, and controlling. The effectiveness of these activities can be determined by assessing various structures, processes, and outcomes in the environment. This chapter will suggest the types of monitors that may be used in six specific functions within the sphere of management:

1. personnel actions
2. budget monitors
3. licensing
4. record keeping and documentation
5. audits on patient charges
6. planning and achieving specific objectives.

By applying the principles demonstrated in each section, a manager can develop monitors for any function in the department.

To obtain a rapid review of management activities from a QA perspective, the manager might find the checklist, published by the American Society of Hospital Pharmacists (ASHP), to be of value.[1] This self-evaluation device has been designed to highlight essential components of a pharmacy's operation. The administrative section covers personnel functions, committee memberships, the policy and procedure manual, and the department's organizational structure. This "mini review" can be expanded to include all facets of departmental operations.

PERSONNEL ACTIONS

One of the most vital concerns of a manager involves the relationships with personnel in the department. Beginning with recruitment and hiring practices, the manager must be certain that anyone hired in a professional position has the required education, skills, and licensure. Tests can be designed to validate the knowledge needed to perform essential functions, both as part of a screening process and as the basis for comparison against later evaluations.

Pharmacy-conducted orientation and in-service training programs are required by the Joint Commission on Accreditation of Hospitals (JCAH) for both nursing and pharmacy personnel. Attendance is to be documented, and the records are to be kept on hand in the department.

Another example of this type of monitoring uses a yearly calendar sheet for each employee. Absences, vacations, holidays, and other similar events can be recorded for reference. Patterns of absenteeism can be detected. This also provides documentation for personnel records. Comparison of absences against preestablished standards will indicate whether counseling or other action may be advisable.

One measure of any employee is the ability to complete assigned tasks within specified time limits; this standard applies to the manager as well. Each institution has required forms and reports, due at specified time intervals. By preparing a chronological checklist of the documents, the manager can ensure that they are completed and submitted on time. This system also permits planning for completion as part of regular duties and assignment of data collection tasks when appropriate.

BUDGET MONITORS

After a department budget is finalized, approved, and implemented, the manager must maintain a system of budget monitors. It is not sufficient to observe where costs or revenues deviate from the budget. The manager must also anticipate and prevent significant discrepancies whenever, and wherever, possible. By working with the hospital's financial officers and the administrator, the manager can develop both a reporting system for receiving pertinent statistical information and a set of standards for measuring actual performance against budgetary expectations.

For example, a ratio between costs and revenue may be established. Each month the actual ratio can be compared with the projected, budgeted ratio and sources of deviation can be identified. In this way, the expenditures remain under control. Some management systems permit semiannual budget adjustments to compensate for either unplanned costs and/or increases in revenue.

Another measurement compares actual labor costs against those costs projected on the budget. The deviations in the calculation may lead to an examination of overtime labor, use of part-time help, and an analysis of the method of distributing the workload over the staffing pattern.

Comparing the current statistics with those of the previous quarter, or year, can also provide the manager with information on trends, such as changes in patient census, increases in labor or drug costs, and impacts of new services on these trends.

The larger the department, the more the manager will have to delegate. The use of monitors on budgetary elements will enable the manager to keep informed and to make changes when needed. When establishing controls, the manager may find it appropriate to use prospective audit techniques to monitor fiscal components.

LICENSING

The pharmacy manager is usually the individual responsible for maintaining current licenses. This means that state and federal licenses must be renewed on time and must be on display. All the pharmacists, however, are responsible for renewing their own respective licenses and for ensuring that they are current and on display in the department.

If sales or tax permits are required, they must also be kept current. Special permits may be required in specific locations. These, too, must also be kept up to date.

Often, the hospital is licensed by the Drug Enforcement Agency (DEA) to order, store, dispense, and administer controlled substances. The pharmacy acts as the agent of the hospital in this case. The license renewal forms will be sent to the hospital administrator for processing, but it is the pharmacist who must ensure that the fee is paid and that the renewal certificate is displayed in the pharmacy.

All of the above items can be included on an annual checklist for the manager. This ensures continuity and documentation for all licensing requirements.

RECORD KEEPING AND DOCUMENTATION

Every aspect of health care requires reams of forms and reports. Pharmacy is no exception. One method that the manager can use to identify required records is to start with two vital documents: the JCAH standards and the policy and procedure manual. Both list the topics that require documentation records. A checklist is useful in fulfilling this requirement. The following is an example of a standard developed to ensure the presence of necessary evidence: All pharmacists must participate in at least 15 hours of continuing education per year, with documentation available in the pharmacy.

Another factor to be determined is the length of storage time. Various records have different storage requirements. Federal and state requirements may also vary. When state and federal storage requirements differ, the longest time period takes precedence. Some of the types of records that must be stored by the pharmacy include:

- prescription files
- patient medication profiles
- Schedule II order blanks, invoices, and perpetual inventory records
- department inventory records
- purchasing records, bid contracts
- personnel files, including applications of those not selected for employment
- equipment maintenance and warranties
- in-service and continuing education records
- minutes of meetings (e.g., pharmacy and therapeutics committee).

Some very real value has been demonstrated for the storage and retrieval of pharmacy records. Two dramatic accounts were published in the *American Journal of Hospital Pharmacy*.[2] A higher than normal incidence of congenital abnormalities was demonstrated in infants of women who had used vaginal spermicides. Prescription records of nine outpatient pharmacies were used to gather data to support this hazard.

The second use of records, mentioned in the same article, involved abuse of an amphetamine capsule. The state of Wisconsin's copies of controlled substance purchase forms were analyzed and revealed that only 5 of the 9,500 licensed practitioners in the state purchased 71 percent of all the doses of the drug in question. Further, it was established that less than 5 percent of Wisconsin pharmacies purchased almost 50 percent of the drug sold to pharmacies. Contacts by licensing boards resulted in decreased usage of the drug, and amphetamine-related arrests increased during the same time period.

The disposal of these mountains of paper also takes some care. First, confidentiality must be maintained. Second, records should not be destroyed prior to the end of the specified storage time but should be isolated and eliminated as soon as possible thereafter. A schedule for removal of old records can be established and responsible individuals given these tasks. Since space is at a premium, the value of the prompt removal of old records is easily demonstrable. With the advent of the use of computers in many hospitals, files are stored and retrieved electronically. The efficiency of this method cannot be underestimated. A back-up system (manual) may be required in the event of computer breakdown. Confidentiality also must be maintained when records are stored in a computer.

AUDITS ON PATIENT CHARGES

A time-consuming task is the verification of charges on a patient's bill. If a concurrent monitoring process samples and verifies patients' pharmacy charges, it is possible to locate and correct error sources. For example, a specific number of discharge bills could be examined each day. By recording the type and frequency of errors, the accuracy in billing can be determined.

Another source of this type of data is generated by late charges (i.e., those added to the bill after the patient has been discharged). Since this is an undesirable fiscal procedure, the number of late charges should be kept below a preestablished amount. Identifying causes of late charges may lead to a multidisciplinary problem-solving exercise (e.g., a delay in charges turned in to pharmacy from respiratory therapy slowed the completion of discharge billing submitted to the business office). When all of the departments involved worked together to set accepted standards, enforcement of the policy was easier to accomplish.

Certain categories of patients are often subjected to audits by outside agencies (e.g., worker's compensation patients). If this becomes a standard practice in the institution, it might be wise to perform a discharge verification of all charges on the bills of worker's compensation patients. This "ounce of prevention" can save a substantial amount of time and money later if the chart and bill are audited.

Another area for periodic monitoring by the manager could be the prices being charged for outpatient medications. This category includes take-home medications, emergency room prescriptions, drugs sold to hospital employees and medical staff, and clinic prescriptions. Comparison of prices on the prescription file, against established charging policies, will provide easily obtainable data. It is often true that each pharmacist applies the formula in a slightly different manner. An in-service or counseling program may be required to ensure uniform compliance. Again, it is not possible to be certain that "all prescriptions are priced in accordance with established policy" unless this standard is used to measure actual performance.

Other financial areas in the department fall under purchasing and inventory control and are addressed in Chapter 6.

PLANNING AND ACHIEVING SPECIFIC OBJECTIVES

The manager's planning function is one of the most vital in the entire scope of activities. All other members of a department carry out tasks to achieve predetermined goals. The setting of goals and charting of the course to achieve them is accomplished by the manager. David Campbell has been quoted as saying, "If you don't know where you're going, you'll probably wind up someplace else!"[3]

Management by objectives (MBOs) and performance evaluation review techniques (PERT) are two of the methods used by managers to plan for the attainment of goals. Further, the achievement of these goals within the allotted time periods is a measure of the effectiveness of a manager.

The subjects of both specific objectives and quality assurance fit together like a lock and key. Quality assurance helps the manager identify problems as opportunities for growth and change. The objective of the process of change is the goal set by the department manager. The action plan will lead participants to the desired results. Quality assurance will verify that the original problem has been solved. Reevaluation will ensure that it continues to remain an effective solution. One of the most gratifying aspects of quality assurance is its strength as a tool to assist the manager in unlocking the door leading to the achievement of planned objectives.

For quality assurance to be of practical value, it should be used to identify and help to solve problems. Golightly, in her book *Creative Problem Solving for Health Care Professionals,* states that problem solving consumes a significant portion of a health care manager's day.[4] Therefore, quality assurance can be used as a device to ensure that identified problems are resolved quickly and efficiently.

NOTES

1. "Two-Minute Self-Evaluation of the Status of Your Pharmacy Service," in *Model Quality Assurance Program for Hospital Pharmacies* (Washington, D.C.: American Society of Hospital Pharmacists, 1978).

2. "What Good Are Pharmacy Records?" *American Journal of Hospital Pharmacy* 38 (1981): 1103.

3. David Campbell, *If You Don't Know Where You're Going, You'll Probably Wind Up Someplace Else* (Niles, Ill.: Argus Communications, 1974).

4. Cecilia K. Golightly, *Creative Problem Solving for Health Care Professionals* (Rockville, Md.: Aspen Systems Corp., 1981).

Chapter 11

Professional Interactions

11

The most effective committee is made up of three men, two of whom are absent.

—*Sir Herbert Beerbohm Tree*

Working in a hospital has been compared with living in a small town. Few significant events take place without everyone knowing about and being affected by them. It is important to keep this concept in mind when planning, implementing, or monitoring any health care activity. It is rare that a change in a policy or procedure will not produce ramifications outside the department originating the alteration.

To accomplish desired objectives in a hospital, many factors encourage group participation. For example:

- To achieve cooperation of those involved, it is best to invite their assistance at the beginning of a project.
- To obtain desired objectives, hospital organization and management usually encourage committee structures.
- To complete assigned tasks efficiently, it is often advisable to share responsibilities with other individuals.
- To reduce perceived risks, professionals naturally tend to share accountability for suggested changes with peers.
- To foster cooperation among various health professionals, the Joint Commission on Accreditation of Hospitals (JCAH) has purposely designed multidisciplinary requirements within the QA standards.

Duncanis and Golin have defined an interdisciplinary team as a "functioning unit composed of individuals with varied and specialized training, who coordinate their activities to provide services to a client or group of clients."[1] The development of health care teams has been based on the assumption "that an interdisciplinary team will bring together diverse skills and expertise to provide more effective, better coordinated, better quality services for clients."[2]

As hospital pharmacy practice evolved into a discrete entity, more interaction outside the department became necessary. Clinical pharmacy services have further encouraged communication with others in the health care environment. As in other areas of practice discussed in this book, these interprofessional relationships also come under scrutiny through the QA program.

THE PHARMACIST AS A MEMBER OF THE HEALTH CARE TEAM

Hospital bylaws and guidelines from regulatory and professional organizations delineate which committees must include a pharmacist as a member. The traditional requirements include the Pharmacy and Therapeutics Committee, Infection Control Committee, Patient Care Committee, and Safety Committee. Of course, there are several others that the pharmacist may attend by choice or by invitation, such as Quality Assurance, Utilization Review, and other standing committees.

Documentation of participation will certainly include copies of the minutes of each relevant committee. Any pertinent projects or reports, such as drug utilization reviews, should also be attached.

Committees are not the only groups in which the pharmacist works with members of various disciplines; there are many other team efforts in the hospital. Because of the popularity of the team concept, this structure will be examined more closely.

Duncanis and Golin list nine characteristics common to health care teams:[3]

1. A team consists of two or more individuals.
2. The configurations may or may not be face to face.
3. There is an identifiable leader.
4. Teams function within and between organizational settings.
5. Roles of participants are defined.
6. Teams collaborate.
7. There are specific protocols of operation.
8. The team is client (patient) centered.
9. The team is task oriented.

The purpose of conducting an evaluation is to determine which elements of the team approach are effective in a particular setting and which should be eliminated or modified.[4] If evaluation of a team's efforts is required, there are several approaches available. Both concurrent and retrospective assessment techniques are appropriate. Concurrent analysis keeps the program or service "on track," benefiting patients presently receiving it. Retrospective review permits corrections in the future actions of the team, based on documented history. In order to select the appropriate type of analysis, the team will have to evaluate the immediacy of the problem and the desired results of the study efforts.

It may be advisable to look at the *results* of team activities. Can the results be compared with those obtained when the service was not provided by a team? Does the patient benefit more from the use of the team than from other methods of providing the same service? Is it valuable for health care professionals to work together? Does the organization (hospital) benefit (e.g., are communications better)? [5] An instrument for measuring effectiveness can be developed using the questions listed above as a foundation. In addition, there are three other suggested aspects of team performance that can be evaluated:[6]

1. the quality of life for the patient
2. cost effectiveness of the team
3. effectiveness of the team process as an educational medium for team members.

As in other areas of quality assurance, it is also necessary to identify the goals of the service and the indicators that signal achievement of the goals. Without recognition in advance of the desired end point, it is not possible to be sure that the goal has been reached.

When the pharmacist functions as a member of a team or committee, he or she must be aware of the interplay of emotions that takes place, either openly or subliminally. If a conflict develops, it should be examined to find out how and why it happened. The investigation of conflict can uncover hidden problems that might subvert the success of the team's efforts. Once again, the QA process can be applied to the correction of identified problems.

As in any other situation where professionals work closely together, negotiations may be required and "power plays" can be anticipated. It is not appropriate to discuss human relations here, but the reader is encouraged to develop a working knowledge of techniques used for successful negotiation and other related topics. Several books on the subject are recommended at the end of this chapter.

INTRAVENOUS THERAPY TEAMS

One example of a pharmacist functioning on a multidisciplinary team is that of the Intravenous (IV) Therapy Team. Depending on the type of therapy that the patient requires, the pharmacist may be working with nurses, physicians, dietitians, laboratory personnel, physical therapists, radiologists, social workers, and others. It is vital that roles be clearly defined for each team member. Performance evaluation may also be assigned to an interdisciplinary group.

Each aspect of care being rendered should be included in the assessment process—from the initial decisions concerning the patient's therapeutic needs, through the rendering of care, to the ultimate patient outcome. Examples of some of the standards used by IV therapy teams for measuring quality of care are given in Exhibit 11-1.

Exhibit 11-1 Sample QA Standards for Intravenous Therapy Teams

1. Patients' allergies are noted and checked before administration of IV fluids and drugs.

2. All intravenous fluids are administered as prescribed.
   - 2.1 Correct fluids to correct patient.
   - 2.2 Correct rate of administration.
   - 2.3 Correct sequence of fluids.
   - 2.4 Appropriate equipment, e.g., tubing, infusion device.

3. IV tubing is changed routinely, in accordance with the hospital policy (i.e., every 24 or 48 hours).

4. The IV site is rotated every 48-72 hours, in accordance with hospital policy.

5. Documentation for all IV administration site care, tubing and dressing changes, is charted in a timely manner.

Source: HPI Hospital Pharmacies, Inc., Quality Assurance Program for IV Therapy, © 1982. Reprinted with permission.

MONTHLY INSPECTION OF DRUG STORAGE AREAS

Both the JCAH and Medicare standards require that all drug storage areas outside the pharmacy be inspected at least monthly. This includes emergency drug supplies, such as those kept in the crash carts and in the emergency department.[7,8] The inspection should be conducted by members of the pharmacy staff and documented. Copies of inspection reports should be kept on file in the pharmacy and nursing service.

This monthly routine chore can provide opportunities for the alert pharmacist to discuss patient care, to review current medical needs, and to keep the channels of communication open on each nursing unit. These same circumstances also exist in ancillary departments where drugs are stored (e.g., radiology, physical therapy, and other departments). The pharmacist must remember to use tact when inspecting these areas and when filling out the required reports.

Other subjects to be addressed during inspections are lost charges and inventory control. The pharmacist and nursing supervisor should discuss unaccounted for or missing doses to determine causes and to identify, if possible, any needed security or procedural changes. The pharmacist can check on frequency of usage while reviewing the drugs, to ensure that no drug has expired. This procedure may permit reduction in inventory or may highlight areas in which an increase is warranted. Follow-up discussions with supervisors, after inspections are complete, also afford an opportunity for problem solving and other communications between the pharmacist and various health care professionals.

EDUCATIONAL EFFORTS

One more area of interaction involves all the educational programs provided by and for the pharmacy staff. Those individuals who might benefit from such programs outside the department include nursing and medical staff, personnel in ancillary departments, patients, professional pharmacist organizations, and the general community in which the hospital is located.

First, in order to determine the value of educational efforts, it is necessary to establish the needs of the audience with a pretest. Then, after the instructional program has been presented, the effectiveness of the educational material can be measured. A posttest might indicate that the instructor delivered the information efficiently and that the audience received and understood it. After some time has elapsed, the audience can be tested again, to determine whether the information has been retained and used. Analysis of the responses can provide direction for revision of existing material, additional training of the instructor, or development of new programs. Measurement of this type is difficult when programs are offered to the general public, but the information provided by such feedback can be very valuable.

When programs, such as in-service education for hospital personnel are provided, it is advisable to document attendance. Copies should be kept on file, usually by both the provider and the in-service coordinator (if this position exists in the hospital). Each department director who sends staff members to the program should also receive a copy of the record of attendance, since records of educational programs are often examined by inspectors from accrediting and regulatory agencies.

A specialized type of education, patient counseling, should be considered at this time. The same principles used for other educational efforts can also apply here. Several methods have been used to judge the quality of patient counseling programs. Those methods most often used are questionnaires and telephone calls to the patients after they return home.[9]

Evaluation of patient counseling efforts is still a relatively new area for quality assurance. The subject of evaluating clinical pharmacy services in general is thoroughly discussed in Chapter 12.

The provision of drug information services is traditionally assigned to the pharmacy department. The pharmacists who provide this service have yet another opportunity to interact with professionals, students, and the public. Details of QA for drug information services are discussed further in Chapter 12.

It is important to determine that both the medical staff and the hospital administration are aware of the positive feedback to the pharmacy for these educational programs. The QA documentation can be used to demonstrate the value of the pharmacists' efforts toward those individuals receiving them. In the present economic climate in health care, pharmacists must use every tool at their disposal to justify continuation of existing services. One of these tools is the QA program.

ANNUAL REVIEW OF PHARMACY SERVICES BY PHARMACY AND THERAPEUTICS COMMITTEE OR ITS EQUIVALENT

An annual review of pharmacy services by the Pharmacy and Therapeutics Committee (or its equivalent) is required by the JCAH standards.[10] Documentation of the annual review and approval of the policy and procedure manual is usually displayed on the front page of the manual. It is more difficult, however, to document a review of the services provided by the pharmacy. Suggestions are offered for various methods that have been used successfully.

A questionnaire, listing various services for the physician to rate, may be sent to the medical staff. This method has many inherent problems, one being the difficulty of obtaining responses in a timely manner.

Some pharmacists prepare an annual report for the Pharmacy and Therapeutics Committee. Care must be taken to present a balance of both positive and negative factors in the report. Examples of the types of data that may be included in this report are listed below:

- specific objectives, achievements, and obstacles to achievement
- most recent JCAH recommendations and related corrective actions
- review of incident reports, medication error rates, and patient or staff complaints for the previous year
- plans for next year's pharmacy services
- educational programs presented or attended by pharmacy staff
- drug utilization reviews or other studies
- QA activities and results for the previous year

The inclusion of plans for the next year is not usually done in a formal presentation to the committee. Instead, one project at a time is discussed. Both methods have merit. Including plans in the annual review may help reveal pitfalls that can be avoided as each project is actively developed. With the use of this method, a complete picture of departmental activities is then presented for committee approval.

Communication in all directions is vital to the provision of pharmaceutical services in the hospital. Therefore, ensuring the quality of these exchanges of information falls into the realm of the QA program. As in all other phases of health care, efforts expended for QA activities can be used to justify or evaluate interprofessional communications and educational programs provided by pharmacists.

NOTES

1. Alex J. Duncanis and Anne K. Golin, *The Interdisciplinary Health Care Team—A Handbook* (Rockville, Md.: Aspen Systems Corp., 1979), p. 3.
2. Ibid., p. 1.
3. Ibid., pp. 5-7.
4. Ibid., p. 147.
5. Ibid., p. 151.
6. Ibid., p. 145.
7. *Accreditation Manual for Hospitals* (Chicago: Joint Commission on Accreditation of Hospitals, 1981), pp. 138-139.
8. "Conditions for Participation," Medicare Regulations, Department of Health, Education and Welfare, Washington, D.C., 1969, publication no. 19,821, Reg. Sec. 405.1027.

9. Robert L. Kaufman et al., "Medication Discharge Counseling Program Developed by Pharmacists," *Hospitals* 52 (1978): 89-92.

10. *Accreditation Manual for Hospitals*, pp. 137-145.

SUGGESTED READINGS

Berne, Eric. *Games People Play*. New York: Grove Press, 1964.

Cohen, Herb. *You Can Negotiate Anything*. Seacaucus, N.J.: Lyle Stuart, Inc., 1980.

Nierenberg, Gerard I. *Fundamentals of Negotiation*. New York: Hawthorn Books, Inc., 1973.

Chapter 12

Quality Assurance and Clinical Pharmacy Services

Gary L. Snodgrass

12

"It was the best of times, it was the worst of times" wrote Charles Dickens in *A Tale of Two Cities*. In terms of the progress and the future of clinical pharmacy services, this statement could not be more appropriate. Over the past 15 years, the development of clinical pharmacy has occurred at a very rapid rate. Professional pharmacy organizations have acknowledged the importance of this area of practice by devoting numerous committees, task forces, and symposia to study it. In addition, schools of pharmacy are mandated by the American Council of Pharmaceutical Education[1] to include some exposure to clinical pharmacy in their curricula. Textbooks have been published on the subject.[2,3] The federal government has called for increased pharmacist participation in patient education in the form of patient package inserts. Third-party payers are reimbursing some clinical services,[4] and the topic of clinical pharmacy has even been discussed in *Time* magazine.[5] In summary, more than ever before, the pharmacist is in a position to contribute directly to patient care and to have this contribution appreciated by physicians, nurses, administrators, and the public. In this respect, it is the "best of times."

However, a number of variables are simultaneously operating to create a dark cloud on the horizon for clinical pharmacy. New governmental attitudes toward health care funding and prospective reimbursement approaches pose a significant problem for pharmacy administrators. Implementation of new clinical programs or expansion of current ones will be curtailed unless a positive benefit-to-cost ratio can be proved. Capitation funding for pharmacy education is being phased out, and schools are scrambling to determine where future resources to support clinical education and research will come from. Clinical services established as pilot studies, founded on "soft" monies or grants, are facing extinction because of reduced budgets. With so much effort invested, and with the progress of the recent past jeopardized, one could make an argument for the "worst of times."

What panacea can help pharmacy validate the more positive viewpoint? The answer is very simple: evaluation. The systematic and organized evaluation of clinical services is the prime determinant as to whether or not these programs will continue to exist. Obviously this is not a black or white issue. Clinical services will always be offered, either on an individual basis or covertly by certain institutions, regardless of funding. However, to be widely accepted by the public and mandated as a standard of health care practice, clinical services must be funded. The terms *funded* and *evaluated* can almost be used interchangeably. At the very least, the first term should never be used without the latter close behind it, or preferably preceding it. Pharmacy's lack of emphasis on this area in the past is the very reason the "worst of times" concept can even be considered. A pharmacy administrator may not be able to control such ominous variables as health care inflation, but an increased commitment to evaluating department programs is certainly possible.

The purpose of this chapter is to provide a framework for evaluation of clinical services. Basic QA principles outlined throughout this text are also applied to the clinical arena in an effort to quantify, and thus improve, pharmacy's impact on patient care. Before proceeding further the reader is strongly advised to adopt the following assumption: "Quality assurance (evaluation) of clinical services is a necessity, not a luxury."

HISTORY AND DEVELOPMENT

In order to place quality assurance of clinical services in its proper perspective, it is necessary to look briefly at the history of clinical pharmacy in general. The concept was first introduced by Rising in 1945 at the University of Washington and was known as the "Washington experiment."[6] Rising advocated placing pharmacy students in a practice environment for academic credit, but at the time the concept was vigorously disapproved by organized pharmacy.[7] Since the program was quickly discontinued, no evaluation of its impact was reported. However, the seed was planted for expanding the pharmacist's laboratory to the clinical or patient care environment.

Rebirth of the clinical pharmacy concept occurred in the 1960s.[8] Many descriptions of clinical pharmacy were offered, but the only points of commonality were that this new area focused on drug therapy and that it was patient rather than product oriented. From a QA standpoint, the most important historical aspect to concentrate on was a lack of an accepted definition for clinical pharmacy. In addressing the American Society of Hospital Pharmacists in 1967, Parker stated that the term *clinical pharmacy* was "misused and poorly defined." Since in the same speech he proposed that clinical pharmacy "may be either the salvation or the Waterloo for all of Pharmacy," the gravity of this problem is evident.

In 1972, Francke and Whitney wrote: ''Fortunately, no one has yet succeeded in defining clinical pharmacy, and it thus remains an evolving concept with great promise.''[9] Almost 30 years after its introduction, the profession was still struggling with attempts at defining the concept of clinical pharmacy.[10]

Refusing to define a new practice area under the guise of protecting its potential for growth may appear desirable to some. However, this approach is both antithetical to evaluation in general and counterproductive to quality assurance in particular. A cardinal requisite of all QA programs is a clear definition of standards so that accurate measurements of impact can follow. Applied to the development of clinical services, this means that proof of their value was postponed due to a lack of consensus on the exact meaning of clinical pharmacy.

In the 1970s, articles that examined the functions and respective effectiveness of the clinical pharmacist began appearing in the literature.[11-13] Acceptance by physicians of the pharmacists' new role also began to be evaluated.[14-17] Some of the earlier clinical services scrutinized included pharmacist-acquired medication histories[18] and patient discharge counseling.[19] Later reports applied evaluation techniques in order to measure a pharmacist's clinical impact on an ambulatory patient population.[20,21] This interest in role effectiveness quickly spread to measurement of the pharmacist's contribution in disease-specific populations with diabetes,[22] infection,[23] and renal failure.[24] Finally, some attention was given to what often is the most painful topic to research: cost effectiveness.[25-28] Reports range from theoretical projections[29] and philosophical proposals [30] to documented tabulations of third-party reimbursement for clinical services.[31-33] Bibliographies of the pharmacist's cost effectiveness in health care,[34] along with regional surveys of payment for nondistributive (clinical) pharmacy services have also been published.[35]

Several contributions to the literature have established the foundation for a new level of sophistication regarding quality assurance of clinical services. *The Model Quality Assurance Program for Hospital Pharmacies,* published by the American Society of Hospital Pharmacists (ASHP), provides excellent guidance on the development and implementation of an overall pharmacy QA program.[36] Specific clinical services that are briefly discussed include medication histories, discharge counseling, and drug interaction screening. A more in-depth focus on clinical services is offered by Vogel and co-workers.[37] The authors discuss the difference between clinical and distributive pharmacy services and offer several explanations for the lack of growth of clinical QA programs. Among these are inadequate administrative commitment, a relative lack of informal feedback mechanisms to identify clinical program deficiencies, and the fact that clinical pharmacists usually practice independently at a site removed from peer review. The authors proceed to identify 18 minimum standards of pharmacy practice for inpatient care. Seven of these are for clinical services. Audit procedures, exceptions to the standards, and recommended actions for noncompliance are discussed. Both of the above references provide a simplified theoretical framework, along with practical examples, on methods of establishing a QA program for clinical services. More complex evaluation methodology, which can be integrated with these programs, is described in a recent series of articles in *Drug Intelligence and Clinical Pharmacy*.[38-44] The goal of this series is to explore a variety of topics and issues essential to the comprehensive evaluation of clinical programs. One additional indication that progress is being made in the area of clinical services evaluation was the unveiling of a nationwide clinical certification program at the 16th Annual American Society of Hospital Pharmacists Midyear Clinical Meeting.[45,46] This certification effort, designed by HPI Hospital Pharmacies, Inc., encompasses clinical services at over 150 hospitals. It is unique in that methodology is included for quality assurance of both the clinical program and the individual pharmacist's competency.

While it is beyond the scope of this chapter to analyze each of the above references individually, it is possible to identify some general trends in the development of QA programs for clinical services. First and foremost, for a movement identified by some as the "salvation" of the pharmacy profession, there has been an inappropriately small amount of emphasis on evaluation. Considering such strong acceptance on faith from academia, professional organizations, and government, the body of knowledge regarding the impact of clinical services on health care is meager, at best.

A corollary to this trend, again based on historical perspective, is a notable absence of quality as well as quantity of evaluation data. The reader will find that while many of the publications on clinical services have merit, only a few employ sound experimental design. The necessity of using randomization, blinding, controls, and statistical analysis becomes obvious when one considers the variety of people assessing the study. One clinical pharmacist may accept on faith a significant amount of hypothesis from another because both of their value systems and frames of reference are similar. However, it should be kept in mind that clinical services are evaluated daily by a diverse population of physicians, nurses, patients, and hospital administrators, as well as by individuals in government and private industry. If a lesson can be taken from the past, not only do clinical pharmacists need to adopt a stronger stance on quantifying their impact, but every attempt should be made to strengthen the accuracy and precision of the measuring process. One final trend, woven throughout the history of the evaluation of clinical programs, is more subtle. Although it is difficult to generalize, the extent of evaluation seems dependent on the organizational position of the person responsible for the evaluation process. In those instances where clinicians providing the service were also totally responsible for its evaluation, the tendency has been to collect less data. A number of explanations for this include conflict of interest, inadequate resources, lack of evaluation expertise, insufficient time, and human nature. Most clinicians, pressed with the choice of either providing patient care or doing evaluative research, rarely opt for the latter. This helps explain the plethora of patient case reports and descriptive publications on clinical services relative to the small number of evaluation studies that have been authored by clinicians. As the role of evaluator began to be filled by academician/researchers, the amount of clinical program assessment data in the literature increased. The most recent step in this continuum has been the assumption of evaluator-responsibility by pharmacy administrators. In those instances where the director of pharmacy has taken an active part in evaluation planning, the growth and success of QA programs for clinical services have accelerated.

The purpose of developing this line of reasoning is to prevent the reader from succumbing to the trap historically fallen into by many pharmacy administrators. It is a myth for an administrator to believe that, because he or she does not understand pharmacokinetics, it follows that he or she should not be involved in evaluating clinical services. Working in concert with the clinician, the director should help map out the goals and objectives of evaluation, budget the necessary resources, plan the methodology, and design the milestone chart or timetable for results. This approach injects administrative expertise and in-hospital political clout into the QA program. In addition, it clearly communicates to the pharmacy staff that evaluation is a priority; it also conveys to others in the hospital that the pharmacy is willing to take an objective look at its own services.

A BASIC PARADIGM FOR QUALITY ASSURANCE

There are many excellent treatises on the basics of QA theory; therefore, for detail, the reader is referred to Chapter 3 of this text and to the work of others.[47] What follows is a distillation of these works to emphasize application, as opposed to theory. A simplified introduction to quality assurance can be envisioned as a five-step process:

1. Define what is to be measured and establish standards.
2. Measure it.
3. Attempt to change the "real" in step 2 to conform to the "ideal" in step 1.
4. Measure it again.
5. Compare the results in step 4 with the reasonableness of the standards in step 1 and redefine if necessary. Periodically update the standards.

Another paraphrase of this five-step process is offered by Horowitz and Lamnin:[48]

1. Define quality (standards, criteria).
2. Assess performance.

3. Determine compliance to standards and take necessary corrective action.
4. Reassess performance.
5. Redefine quality.

A more graphic expansion of this model is presented in Figure 12-1. Definitions of key terms used in the model in Figure 12-1 are as follows:

- *Criteria* are written statements, against which aspects of the quality of a service can be measured.[49]

Figure 12-1 ASHP QA Process Model

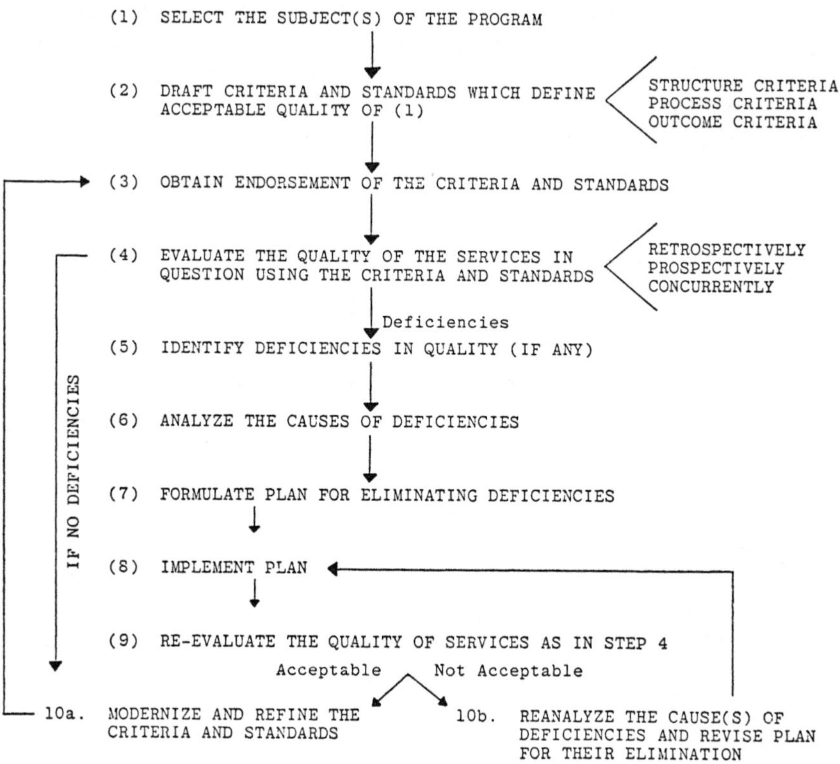

Source: Adapted, with permission, from the *Model Quality Assurance Program for Hospital Pharmacies* published by the American Society of Hospital Pharmacists.

- *Standards* define the amount of acceptable deviation from a criterion. Standards are the form in which criteria are used to evaluate a given subject.[50]
- *Structure* criteria refer to the resources, facilities, and organization of the pharmacy department or individual providing the product or service.[51]
- *Process criteria* refer to the procedures that are considered necessary to provide an acceptable product or service.[52]
- *Outcome criteria* refer to the results of a service or direct observation of a finished product.[53]

Several points should be kept in mind when applying any QA model to clinical services. First, it is not necessary to create a separate model for clinical services. The basic principles of quality assurance apply whether or not a product is produced or a service is rendered. Often the two are so closely intertwined in pharmacy that a firm distinction between clinical and distributive services is impossible. Instead, one should think in terms of the component functions of the overall service. How many tasks are patient oriented (clinical) and how many are product oriented (distributive)? This analysis of emphasis will help select the type of criteria needed for meaningful quality assurance. A second, closely related principle advocates that one adjust the type of criteria used to match both the environment and the subject to be measured. In general, whenever possible, it is desirable to use outcome criteria. However, the complexity of a clinical service may make measurement of outcomes impractical. For example, it may not be possible to distinguish whether a patient's response is due to the application of the therapy or to the normal progression of the disease. In these instances, the QA program may be forced to emphasize process rather than outcome criteria. Similarly, if the service to be measured involves furnishing drug information, a greater emphasis on structure criteria (resources) may be appropriate. In summary, the basic steps of a QA model should remain uniform when evaluating different services. Only the specifics of emphasis need be adjusted to meet the unique goals and methodology of the clinical service.

One final principle involves the frequency of evaluation. Although data analysis will be done periodically, evaluation data for clinical services should be collected continuously. It is desirable that quality assurance of clinical services be ongoing or continuous, rather than periodic. The importance of this principle lies in the serious patient consequences that may result from discontinuous evaluation. For example, substandard quality may go unrecognized for weeks or months if only periodic evaluation is used. Another consideration is that state-of-the-art knowledge of clinical services is changing more rapidly than that of distributive services. In any service where obsolescence of method is a significant danger, the need for ongoing quality assurance is intensified.

APPLICATION OF THE QA MODEL TO DRUG INFORMATION SERVICES

Possession of accurate drug information is a prerequisite for virtually every therapeutic decision made by the clinical pharmacist. With the rapid search, retrieval, and interpretation of information on drugs occupying such a high priority in clinical services, it is worthwhile to give special attention to quality assurance for this area. At the same time, it is surprising to note that many formal drug information centers do not have an organized QA program to measure their impact.

The provision of drug information can be considered a clinical service in that the primary function involved is interpretation of facts to provide advice. This advice or consultation may directly or indirectly affect patient care. The sophistication of drug information services spans a continuum, from a single pharmacist responding to a physician's inquiry concerning the color of diazepam (Valium) 10-mg tablets to a thorough literature search on the potential of erythromycin estolate causing hepatotoxicity in children. The example below illustrates the application of steps, delineated in Figure 12-1, to a formal drug information center (DIC) at a medium-sized hospital. However, the sophistication of the model can be adjusted up or down to fit drug information services falling anywhere along the continuum.

Step 1—Select the Subjects of the Program

What services or functional areas will the program cover? Will answering patient-specific questions, doing literature searches, and providing copies of actual articles be covered? Do services, such as writing reports to the Pharmacy and Therapeutics Committee or participation in investigational drug research projects, need to be included in the QA program? All the major functions of the drug information center should be listed and prioritized with reference to their need to be measured.

Step 2—Draft Criteria and Standards That Define Acceptable Quality

When each major function of the drug information center has been selected for measurement, criteria for performance excellence should be written. For example, structure criteria could include: "The drug information center is open from 8:00 A.M. to 10:00 P.M. every day, with a pharmacist on call the remaining time," or "A good reference library is available." An example of a standard to measure the latter criteria might be: "At least two of the following drug information retrieval systems (e.g., Iowa, DeHaen, Drugdex) are located in the DIC." To digress, this same approach could be used by the individual pharmacist interested in applying quality assurance to the pharmacy's provision of drug information. A sample standard for structure criteria would be: "Personal files contain 90 percent of the reference articles recommended in *Therapeutics Bibliography for Clinical Pharmacists*."[54] Other core references are suggested for either the individual or the hospital library to expand this concept.[55-57]

In addition to structure criteria, process and outcome criteria should be written. Sample process criteria for the drug information center include: "all questions are recorded, including name of caller, time of day, answer given, and references used" and "all responses are checked and co-signed by a registered pharmacist prior to completing the reply." In contrast, outcome criteria could include: "The drug information center averages at least 100 requests per month" and "100 percent of all requests marked STAT are answered within 30 minutes."

It is easy to see that criteria can be designed to serve a variety of needs and consumers. Outcome criteria describing usage rate, as exemplified above, can be presented to administrators to justify the cost/benefit of the DIC. The same criteria can be used to determine staffing needs. The point is that rational judgments on these issues cannot be made without well-defined and appropriate QA criteria and standards. They certainly cannot be made without any QA program at all. Due to the wide variation in drug information center goals and resources, the reader is strongly advised to develop individualized criteria and standards. Further guidance is provided in the literature.[58,59]

Step 3—Obtain Endorsement of the Criteria and Standards

Step 3 refers to the need to double-check the validity of the standards before applying them. One appropriate way of validating the standards is to involve the key individuals or groups in any way affected by the QA process. These people might be simplistically divided into consumers, providers, and accreditors. The accreditors are those that spell out conditions that the service must meet. Therefore, QA standards must conform to their rules. Accreditors include governmental bodies, such as Medicare; voluntary organizations, such as the JCAH; and professional groups, such as the ASHP. For instance, QA criteria for a drug information center may be part of a larger ASHP accreditation of a residency training program.

In a sense, a hospital administrator can also be considered an accreditor, because the DIC must operate within the confines of both the overall hospital policies and procedures and the budget. The administrator should accept the QA criteria, to measure whether or not the center is fulfilling these responsibilities. The second group, that of consumers, will furnish information on the emphasis the service should take. For example, if the drug information center's goal is to serve health professionals in the hospital, then nurses and physicians should have input into the criteria for evaluation. Similarly, input from the providers (those working in the DIC) should help determine if the criteria are fair and practical. In essence, step 3 broadens one's view of the subject to be measured, helps increase commitment from others to the evaluation process, and ensures that the QA standards give fair measurement to the most important aspects of the clinical service.

Step 4—Evaluate the Quality of the Service Using the Criteria and Standards

This phase of the process refers to any differences between actual drug information center practices and the desired criteria/standards. Some thought should be given to the methodology of applying this measurement. It is not enough to have a precision measuring instrument (well-defined standards) if it is applied improperly. First, an evaluator should be chosen who is unbiased but familiar with the standards. Next, it should be decided whether the evaluation will be prospective, concurrent, or retrospective. An example of a prospective approach would be to ask the DIC pharmacist to outline the procedure for handling an emergency poisoning request. A concurrent evaluation might include observation of a request response in progress. Finally, the most common method currently used for quality assurance of drug information centers is retrospective. An annual review of the records of calls summarizes numbers of requests and average time spent per call, for example. This review is desirable in that it focuses on results so that outcome criteria can be applied. However, it should not be the only method applied. Feedback for improving the drug information center service is not frequent enough. Furthermore, inefficiency in the process of handling requests is difficult to diagnose and correct if only outcome criteria are used.

Another consideration in designing the method of evaluation involves selection of the data to be analyzed. In other words, the random sample observations and data collected should be a true reflection of the overall drug information center services to be evaluated. Evaluation should occur at peak hours of activity, as well as at slow times. If the center is not open 24 hours per day, measurements of response time and quality of information should occur for both on-call hours and for normal hours of operation. If possible, observations for process criteria should be made by more than one evaluator to promote greater reliability. The validity of these observations can be improved if the provider does not know when the evaluation is being made. For example, if the evaluator is "looking over the shoulder" of the DIC pharmacist when a request response is being made, the care taken in handling the request may reflect more caution than that used in the normal daily provision of the service. An alternative would be to randomly tape record sample calls. To the reader this amount of effort may seem unwarranted. However, it is not unreasonable, considering that major decisions on budget and expansion or extinction of the DIC could be based on QA results. In addition, a patient's life may depend on the quality of information disseminated by a drug information center. Certainly, the critical nature of the service suggests that a great deal of effort should be invested in the QA process.

Step 5—Identify Deficiencies in Quality (If Any)

All deviation between the observed services and the criteria should be listed in order of importance. Before acting on these deficiencies, the evaluators should agree that the deficiencies are real and not an aberration of the measurement process.

Step 6—Analyze the Causes of the Deficiencies

Previous observation for process criteria can be used here. Resources for the DIC should be analyzed, methodology for responding to requests should be reviewed, and all documentation forms and policies and procedures should be scrutinized.

Step 7—Formulate Plan for Eliminating Deficiencies

The plan should include goals, objectives, methodology, and a timetable. The plan might include budgeting more resources for the center, shifting priorities of service, moving to a new location, or implementing an education and training program for the staff.

Step 8—Implement Plan

Step 9—Reevaluate the Quality of Services

A time frame should be established, based on step 8, allowing adequate time to collect new data reflective of the results of the corrective measures.

Step 10—Modernize or Reanalyze

If the quality of drug information center services now meets the original standards, it may be time to update, redefine, and improve the standards. This last point illustrates the continuous nature of the QA process. Obviously, if deficiencies still exist, new corrective measures must be designed and implemented.

APPLICATION OF THE QA MODEL TO PATIENT-SPECIFIC CLINICAL SERVICES

The same basic steps used to evaluate drug information services can be easily modified to apply quality assurance to patient-specific clinical services. These services include medication histories taken at hospital admission, discharge counseling, patient education, nutritional assessment, parenteral and enteral nutrition consultations, individualized pharmacokinetic dosage adjustments, and several others. An abbreviated illustration, applying the QA model to an aminoglycoside dosing service, is as follows:

Step 1. Assume that the pharmacy at hospital X has been offering aminoglycoside dosing consultations for one year. Services are offered to patients on the sixth and seventh hospital floors only. Subjects of the QA evaluation will include patients over 12 years of age who are receiving tobramycin or amikacin.

Step 2. Sample criteria are written by the pharmacy (Table 12-1). These criteria are not intended to be a comprehensive audit. In a complete QA evaluation, standards would be included to cover peak and trough serum levels, pharmacist reaction to variations in renal function, and a host of other factors. Other criteria of a nonclinical nature could include "Physicians implemented pharmacy dosing recommendations at least 90 percent of the time" or "Over 50 percent of the physicians prescribing aminoglycosides for patients on floors six and seven requested pharmacy consultations."

Step 3. Criteria were presented to the hospital Pharmacy and Therapeutics Committee and to the Infection Control Committee. Both of these committees approved all criteria but revised the QA evaluation to include gentamicin. A decision was also made to include a minimum of 50 patients in the audit.

Step 4. Pharmacy profiles were reviewed to identify all sixth and seventh floor patients given the selected aminoglycoside over the past three months. Charts were retrieved from medical records, and data were collected retrospectively. Only 27 patients meeting study criteria were identified. Concurrent data were then collected for the next 23 patients meeting the selection criteria. This last step took an additional two months.

Step 5. Major deficiencies included a failure to record weight in 68 percent of patients and serum creatinine in first 24 hours 40 percent of the time.

Step 6. Analysis of deficiencies revealed that the responsibility for recording a patient's weight was not clearly assigned to anyone in particular. Some physicians did not acknowledge the importance of a baseline serum creatinine measurement and did not routinely order it. Also, patients admitted in the

Table 12-1 Sample Criteria for an Aminoglycoside Dosing Service

CRITERIA	IDEAL STANDARD	ACTUAL % FOUND	EXCEPTION	DATA SOURCE
1. Patient parameters are:				
1.1 Age	100%		None	Admission info.
1.2 Actual weight	100%		None	Admission info.
1.3 Ideal body weight	100%		None	Reference text
1.4 Height	100%		None	Admission info.
1.5 Sex	100%		None	Admission info.
2. Total daily initial dose based on ideal body weight not to exceed:				
2.1 5mg/kg/day for Tobramycin	100%		None, unless previously documented patient idiosyncratic need for higher doses of aminoglycosides	Physician's order sheet in chart, Pharmacy profiles
2.2 15mg/kg/day for Amikacin	100%			
2.3 Two grams total dosage/day based on ideal body weight	100%			
3. Serum creatinine is drawn within 24 hours of the initiation of therapy.	100%		None	Lab reports in chart

afternoon were sometimes missed, because the laboratory personnel normally drew serum samples in the morning.

Step 7. Corrective action might include design of a written protocol regarding methods of following therapy for aminoglycoside patients. The nursing staff could be assigned sole responsibility for obtaining weights for all patients. All physicians' orders for aminoglycosides could be accompanied by an automatic STAT order for serum creatinine. In addition, pharmacy could present an in-service lecture on aminoglycosides, in general, and the importance of the above functions, in particular.

The reader should be able to devise steps 8 through 10 independently to complete this illustration.

QUALITY ASSURANCE AND PROFESSIONAL COMPETENCE

One of the most confusing and controversial aspects of clinical practice is the evaluation of professional competence. Since judgments are being passed on an individual's performance rather than on a program, this topic is characteristically charged with emotion. Adding to this is the fact that there is little agreement among educational researchers on an exact method of measuring competence. In addition, if agreement among educators is scarce, consensus among clinical practitioners is nonexistent! For example, in 1976 the American Board of Medical Specialties adopted guidelines for practitioner recertification, stating that "all member boards shall consider the implementation of a recertification process in the reasonably near future." Four years later only 5 of 23 boards had conducted recertification programs.[60] An editorial[61] on the subject of recertification brought some of the following comments from physicians:

- "Written examinations . . . are totally inadequate for recertification."[62]
- "There is no testing mechanism that can guarantee competence."[63]
- "Incompetent physicians will expose their ineptness. We are fast becoming a generation of examination heroes."[64]

Since the profession of medicine has the longest history of experience with practitioner certification, it is not difficult to extrapolate, from this history, the lack of agreement on the topic. Most of the literature in this area describes clinical performance evaluation of students, rather than evaluation of practitioners. For background reading concerning the evaluation of students in various health professions, please refer to the suggested readings at the end of this chapter.

Several articles that specifically focus on the clinical performance of pharmacy practitioners have appeared in the literature. Mannone describes the use of minimum standard examinations to ensure staff competency and evaluate job performance.[65] Schneider and associates propose a competency-based advancement program for pharmacists, employing a number of QA structure criteria to decide promotion and salary levels.[66] Burkle and co-workers have developed competency standards for quality assurance in clinical pharmacokinetics.[67] However, most references still approach the assessment of practitioner performance only indirectly. For example, despite the title, "The Quality Assurance of Professional Staff," Vogel and associates really describe *program* rather than *practitioner* evaluation.[68]

In the midst of all this sophisticated disagreement, how can one begin to approach the issue of professional competency? One alternative is to try some practical modification of the basic QA model. The same basic principles will work if human nature is kept in mind and if it is accepted that assessment of individuals is likely to be perceived as a threat. In addition, the evaluator must have significant resources at his or her disposal because of the complexity and resultant cost involved.

As before, the first step should be to select the subject of the evaluation. This step should be expanded to answer all of the following questions: Who is to be evaluated? What practice areas are to be examined? For what purposes will the data be used? What effect will both the evaluation process and the results have on the practitioners? Pharmacists are more likely to cooperate and increase the validity of the QA process if it is diagnostic and formative, rather than if evaluation is summative and judgmental.

The second step is to define criteria and standards. Before this can be accomplished for any one clinical service, some common ground has to be reached on the definition of the term *competence*. For the purpose of this discussion, it is proposed that competence be defined as "the appropriate translation of knowledge into action." Therefore, clinical competence can be defined as the use of knowledge and judgment to demonstrate skill in caring for patients effectively. These simple definitions allow the evaluator to design measurable criteria for clinical performance. It is not enough to possess only knowledge. The competent clinician must translate knowledge into appropriate action, and actions can be measured. For purposes of illustration, *Bloom's Taxonomy of Educational Objectives* can be used.[69,70] Bloom categorizes learning into the domains of cognitive, affective, and psychomotor skills. Demonstration of competence must draw upon all three. Therefore, evaluation of competence must include measurement strategies to collect data from all three domains.

The clinical service involving a pharmacist's response to cardiopulmonary arrest codes can be used as an example. The pharmacist's clinical competence depends on knowledge of the appropriate drug and its correct dose for the treatment of various arrhythmias. This knowledge draws from the cognitive domain, and although it is a prerequisite to competence, this knowledge by itself does not positively impact patient care. The pharmacist must have the affective skill to be confident enough under pressure to offer this information. Similarly, psychomotor skills must be present to enable accurate preparation and measurement of the dose, once the physician's order is given. The implications of this concept in designing a QA program for pharmacists participating in cardiopulmonary resuscitation services are obvious. Measurement of competence will require more than design of a multiple choice test on doses and side effects. The observation of actual performance is necessary. With these points in mind, the evaluator can establish the criteria and standards for each clinical service or skill. A task analysis of the role of the pharmacist and the specific functions to be performed will facilitate this.

Endorsement of the criteria can be accomplished by reviewing the literature for standards of practice, by discussion of the appropriateness of the standards among the pharmacy staff, and by presentation to various multidisciplinary committees, such as the Pharmacy and Therapeutics Committee. Since problem solving or clinical judgment occurs in widely differing patterns or sequences among clinicians, outcome criteria should be used whenever possible. When process criteria must be resorted to it is even more important to spend time gaining consensus on the fairness of the standards before applying them. The QA process is likely to meet with strong resistance if a clinician senses that the thinking process itself is under a microscope or that judgment may be questioned.

Finally, it is important to stress that, although routinely used to predict competence, structural criteria are the most unreliable. Possession of certain academic degrees or of a given number of years' experience is often used as the only criterion for estimating competence. Competence is not a static commodity, and, therefore, it may deteriorate with time. Inferring clinical competence from structural criteria is ill advised.

The next step in the QA process is to evaluate the clinician's actual performance, using the predetermined criteria and standards. The principles outlined previously for quality assurance programs also apply to quality assurance for practitioners:

- Select an unbiased evaluator.
- Decide whether evaluation will be prospective, concurrent, or retrospective.
- Sample evaluation data randomly.
- Ensure that data represent the entire universe of clinical functions performed by the practitioner.
- Consider the context of the evaluation.

With reference to the last point concerning the context of evaluation, it must be decided whether the clinician will be evaluated in the context of his or her normal daily activities or will the evaluation take place at a preselected time, with all conditions controlled? Either choice may be appropriate, depending upon the purpose of the evaluation.

For example, a director of pharmacy wishes to begin an aminoglycoside dosing program. However, only the resources to commit one full-time equivalent staff member to the task for three months are available. Twelve of 15 staff members volunteer, and structure criteria are used to screen out all but five people. In this instance, the administrator is trying to choose the most competent person, but the evaluation must be made on ability rather than habitual performance. In essence, individual competence is being judged on a prospective basis. Therefore, a performance test on aminoglycoside kinetics, in which all extraneous variables are held constant, is justified.

In contrast, assume that the director was trying to select, for a merit increase, the most competent practitioner from among five pharmacists who have been offering aminoglycoside dosing consultations for the past three months. Here the evaluation of habitual performance is preferable to that of raw ability. Rather than a performance test with all variables held constant, the evaluation should include naturalistic observations. This means that the evaluation will occur in the context of the pharmacist's daily activities and that observations will be made on the wards or while the clinical service is being provided. Both situations deal with quality assurance of professional competence. However, the purpose of the evaluation may dictate an entirely different approach.

The remaining steps of the basic QA model should be familiar enough to the reader so that they can now be applied to individual competence. However, step 7, that of formulating a plan to correct deficiencies, deserves special mention. It is strongly recommended that any plan for corrective action be individualized carefully for each pharmacist. Learning styles may differ; therefore, a lecture format for communicating new knowledge is suitable for one person, whereas independent study may produce better results in another.

A pharmacist's self-image and ability to accept criticism will strongly influence the design of the corrective plan. Negotiated goal setting with management, accompanied by a timetable for acquiring clinical skills, may be suitable. Peer group feedback and evaluation may help one pharmacist remove deficiencies, yet may prove an impediment to another. Lack of practitioner confidence may necessitate role-playing methodology or the use of "mock" clinical situations to reduce anxiety when later approaching real patients. Following this line of thinking, there are a myriad of considerations that should be evaluated for inclusion in any plan to correct deficiencies in individual clinical performance. In summary, the plan should be constructive, supportive, and practical; contain both positive and negative feedback; and have a negotiated time frame for achieving performance goals.

SUMMARY

The following summary statements provide the reader with an overview of quality assurance of clinical services:

- Quality assurance of clinical services is a necessity and should be an integral part of all clinical programs.
- Pharmacy administrators should play an active role in any QA program that includes quality assurance of clinical services.
- QA principles can be used to design a basic model applicable to both distributive and clinical services.
- The measurable criteria used in a QA program should be matched to the environment and the subject to be assessed.
- A QA program for clinical services should emphasize outcome criteria, but, in general, these should not be the only type of criteria used.
- Evaluation data for clinical services should be collected continuously, and quality assurance should be applied on an ongoing basis.
- Endorsement of criteria and standards, by key individuals, is a crucial step in applying quality assurance to clinical services.
- Quality assurance for clinical services should include both evaluation of program effectiveness and practitioner competence.
- A clear definition of competence, along with consensus among the evaluators, is essential to the success of quality assurance for practitioners.
- Clinical competence is not a static commodity; therefore, it may deteriorate with time. As with quality assurance for programs, quality assurance for practitioners should be ongoing, in the form of recertification.
- Quality assurance of practitioners requires that the context of evaluation also be considered.
- All corrective plans for eliminating practitioner deficiencies should be carefully individualized.
- The application of quality assurance to professional competence should use sound management principles, make optimal use of formal and informal feedback mechanisms, and include a negotiated time frame for achieving performance goals. Above all, it should be constructive, supportive and practical, and set high goals for quality in patient care.

NOTES

1. *Accreditation Manual, 7th ed.: Policy, Procedure and Standards to be Used as the Basis for Accreditation of Programs of Colleges of Pharmacy* (Chicago: The American Council on Pharmaceutical Education, January 1, 1975).

2. Donald E. Francke & Whitney, eds., *Perspectives in Clinical Pharmacy* (Hamilton, Ill.: Drug Intelligence Publications, 1972).

3. Charles W. Blissitt, Lynn O. Webb, and Walter F. Stanaszek, *Clinical Pharmacy Practice* (Philadelphia: Lea & Febiger, 1972).

4. Fred R. Curtiss, "Reimbursement for Clinical Pharmacy Services," *Topics in Hospital Pharmacy Management* 2, no. 1 (1982): 6-21.

5. "More than Just Pill Counters," *Time*, October 12, 1981, p. 95.

6. H.W. Youngken, Jr., "The Washington Experiment—Clinical Pharmacy," *American Journal of Pharmaceutical Education* 17 (1953): 64-70.

7. H.S. Johnson, chairman, "Report of the Committee on Educational and Membership Standards," *American Journal of Pharmaceutical Education* 10 (1946): 80-90.

8. Francke & Whitney, *Perspectives in Clinical Pharmacy*, p. 26.

9. Ibid., p. vii.

10. F. Eshelman, "Clinical Pharmacy Defined," *Drug Intelligence and Clinical Pharmacy* 9 (1975): 688.

11. W.A. Miller, "Selection, Training, and Evaluation of Clinical Pharmacists," *American Journal of Hospital Pharmacy* 31 (1974): 448.

12. A.A. Nelson, Jr., et al., "Task Analysis of a Pharmacist's Activities in a 45-Bed Rural Hospital with Comprehensive Pharmaceutical Services," *American Journal of Hospital Pharmacy* 34 (1977): 1063.

13. D.J. Tanner, "Comprehensive Pharmaceutical Services in an 85-Bed Hospital: A One-Year Evaluation," *American Journal of Hospital Pharmacy* 34 (1977): 486.

14. G.G. Briggs and W.E. Smith, Jr., "Pharmacist-Physician Consultations in a Community Hospital," *American Journal of Hospital Pharmacy* 31 (1974): 247.

15. J.E. Bell, V.E. Bouchard, J.C. South, and M.G. Duffy, "A New Approach to Delivering Drug Information to the Physician Through a Pharmacy Consultation Program—Evaluation Methodology," *American Journal of Hospital Pharmacy* 30 (1973): 220 and 300.

16. A.A. Nelson, Jr., J.M. Meinhold, and R.A. Hutchinson, "Changes in Physician's Attitudes Toward Pharmacists as Drug Information Consultants Following Implementation of Clinical Pharmaceutical Services," *American Journal of Hospital Pharmacy*, 35 (1978): 1201.

17. J.H. Hull and F.M. Eckel, "Evaluation of the Pharmacist as a Drug Therapy Advisor on Ward Rounds," *American Journal of Hospital Pharmacy* 30 (1973): 687.

18. R.S. Wilson and H.F. Kabat, "Pharmacist-Initiated Patient Drug Histories," *American Journal of Hospital Pharmacy* 28 (1971): 45.

19. P. Cole and Sister Emmanuel, "Drug Consultation: Its Significance to the Discharged Hospital Patient and its Relevance as a Role for the Pharmacist," *American Journal of Hospital Pharmacy* 28 (1971): 954.

20. D.K. Solomon et al., "Use of Medication Profiles to Detect Potential Therapeutic Problems in Ambulatory Patients," *American Journal of Hospital Pharmacy* 31 (1974): 348.

21. C.A. Sczupak and W.F. Conrad, "Relationship Between Patient-Oriented Pharmaceutical Services and Therapeutic Outcomes of Ambulatory Patients with Diabetes Mellitus," *American Journal of Hospital Pharmacy* 34 (1977): 1238.

22. Ibid.

23. Scott Davis, "Evaluation of Pharmacist Management of Streptococcal Throat Infections in a Health Maintenance Organization," *American Journal of Hospital Pharmacy* 35 (1978): 561.

24. V.A. Skoutakis et al., "Role-Effectiveness of the Pharmacist in the Treatment of Hemodialysis Patients," *American Journal of Hospital Pharmacy* 35 (1978): 62.

25. G. Marshall, "Clinical Program May Effect Savings," *Hospitals* 48 (1974): 79.

26. M.R. Cohen, S.J. Turco, and A.J. Weltman, "An Assessment of the Impact and Value of Clinical Pharmacy Services," *Hospital Pharmacy* 12 (1977): 9.

27. F.R. Barsness and C.E. Trinca, "Activity Analysis and Cost Study of Clinical Pharmacists Practicing in a University Medical Center," *Drug Intelligence and Clinical Pharmacy* 12 (1978): 284.

28. W.F. McGhan, C.R. Rowland, and J.L. Bootman, "Cost-Benefit and Cost-Effectiveness: Methodologies for Evaluating Innovative Pharmaceutical Services," *American Journal of Hospital Pharmacy* 35 (1978): 133.

29. D.M. Stuart, "Cost Benefits of Clinical Pharmacy," *Drug Intelligence and Clinical Pharmacy* 10 (1976): 181.

30. D.J. Tanner, "A Fee for the Service of Pharmacy: The Time Has Come," *Hospital Pharmacy* 13 (1978): 692.

31. L.E. Patterson and R.J. Huether, "Reimbursement for Clinical Pharmaceutical Services," *American Journal of Hospital Pharmacy* 35 (1978): 1373.

32. W.E. Smith and J.W. Weiblen, "Charging for Hospital Pharmaceutical Services: Product Cost, Per Diem Fees and Fees for Special Clinical Services," *American Journal of Hospital Pharmacy* 36 (1979): 355.

33. E.G. Nold and D.S. Pathak, "Third-Party Reimbursement for Clinical Pharmacy Services: Philosophy and Practice," *American Journal of Hospital Pharmacy* 34 (1977): 823.

34. I. Rubin, "These 19 Statistical Studies Prove Pharmacists' Cost-Effectiveness in Health," *Pharmacy Times*, December 1978, p. 46.

35. L.R. Strandberg, D.J. Stennett, and W. Simonson, "Payment for Nondistributive Hospital Pharmacy Services—A Regional Survey," *Drug Intelligence and Clinical Pharmacy* 12 (1978): 410.

36. *Model Quality Assurance Program for Hospital Pharmacies* (Washington, D.C.: American Society of Hospital Pharmacists, 1978).

37. D.P. Vogel, E. Gurwich, and R.A. Hutchinson, "The Quality Assurance of Professional Staff," *Current Concepts in Hospital Pharmacy Management*, Summer 1981, pp. 8-17.

38. D.S. Pathak, "Evaluation of Clinical Programs: An Operational Framework," *Drug Intelligence and Clinical Pharmacy* 15 (1981): 459.

39. A. Fink and J. Kosecoff, "Evaluating Clinical Programs: Methodological Guidelines," *Drug Intelligence and Clinical Pharmacy* 15 (1981): 536.

40. W.F. McGhan, "Dilemmas in Evaluating Health Care and Clinical Programs," *Drug Intelligence and Clinical Pharmacy* 15 (1981): 684.

41. K.N. Lohr and R.H. Brook, "Quality Assurance and Clinical Pharmacy: Lessons From Medicine," *Drug Intelligence and Clinical Pharmacy* 15 (1981): 758.

42. J.E. Ware, Jr., "How to Survey Patient Satisfaction," *Drug Intelligence and Clinical Pharmacy* 15 (1981): 892.

43. A. Fink and J. Kosecoff, "Needs Assessment: Selecting Clinical Goals," *Drug Intelligence and Clinical Pharmacy* 15 (1981): 986.

44. M. Scriven, "Needs Assessment," *Drug Intelligence and Clinical Pharmacy* 16 (1982): 56.

45. R. Talley, "Certification Program for Clinical Services Developed by HPI Hospital Pharmacies," editorial, *American Journal of Hospital Pharmacy* 38 (October 1981): 1418 and 1420.

46. Gary L. Snodgrass et al., "Implementation of Clinical Services in a Multihospital System," Management Case Study, American Society of Hospital Pharmacists Midyear Clinical Meeting, December 1981.

47. *Model Quality Assurance Program for Hospital Pharmacies.*

48. Kenneth N. Horowitz and Marlene Lamnin, "Design and Implementation of a Quality Assurance Program for Pharmaceutical Services," *American Journal of Hospital Pharmacy* 37 (January 1980): 82-84.

49. *Model Quality Assurance Program for Hospital Pharmacies,* p. 5.

50. Ibid.

51. W.A. Miller, "Quality Assurance of Pharmacy Services," in *The Practice of Pharmacy* (Cincinnati: Harvey Whitney Books, 1981), p. 376.

52. Ibid.

53. Ibid.

54. A.W. Rosman, "Therapeutics Bibliography for Clinical Pharmacists," *American Journal of Hospital Pharmacy* 37 (1980): 406.

55. W.J. Tomasulo, "Core References for the Hospital Pharmacy Library," *Hospital Formulary* 13, no. 10, October 1978, p. 793.

56. J.L. Hirschman, "Building a Clinically Oriented Drug Information Service," in *Perspectives in Clinical Pharmacy*. Donald E. Franke, ed. (Hamilton, Ill.: Drug Intelligence Publications, 1972).

57. *Information Sources for Pharmacists* (Washington, D.C.: American Pharmaceutical Association Foundation Library, 1978).

58. G.J. Merritt, W.R. Garnett, and F.M. Eckel, "Analysis of a Hospital Based Drug Information Center," *American Journal of Hospital Pharmacy* 34 (1977): 43.

59. G.H. Smith, chairman, *Guidelines for Quality Assurance for Drug Information Services* (Washington, D.C.: American Society of Hospital Pharmacists Special Interest Group on Drug and Poison Information Practice, 1980).

60. G.R. Leymaster, "Recertification: Will We Retreat?" *New England Journal of Medicine* 302 (1980): 411.

61. A.S. Relman, "Recertification: Will We Retreat?" *New England Journal of Medicine* 301 (1979): 778.

62. I.D. Fagin, Letter, *New England Journal of Medicine* 302 (1980): 411.

63. J.K. Freedman, Letter, *New England Journal of Medicine* 302 (1980): 411.

64. I.F. Norstrand, Letter, *New England Journal of Medicine* 302 (1980): 411.

65. L.J. Mannone, "Competency of Pharmacy Staff Tested, Fostered," *Hospitals*, December 1980, p. 77.

66. P.J. Schneider et al., "Competency-Based Advancement Program for Pharmacists," *American Journal of Hospital Pharmacy* 38 (1981): 1331.

67. W.S. Burkle, G.R. Matzke, and R.L. Lucarotti, "Development of Competency Standards for Quality Assurance in Clinical Pharmacokinetics," *Hospital Pharmacy* 15 (1980): 494.

68. Vogel, Gurwich, and Hutchinson, "The Quality Assurance of Professional Staff," pp. 8-17.

69. B. Bloom, *Taxonomy of Educational Objectives, Handbook I: Cognitive Domain* (New York: McKay Company, Inc., 1964).

70. D. Krathwohl, B. Bloom, and B. Masia, *Taxonomy of Educational Objectives, Handbook II: Affective Domain* (New York: McKay Company, Inc., 1964).

SUGGESTED READINGS

Byrne, N., and Cohen, R. "Observational Study of Clinical Clerkship Activities." *Journal of Medical Education* 48 (1973): 922.

Crocker, L.M., et al. "A Performance Rating Scale for Evaluating Clinical Competence of Occupational Therapy Students." *American Journal of Occupational Therapy* 29 (1975): 81.

Graham, J.R. "Systematic Evaluation of Clinical Competence." *Journal of Medical Education* 46 (1971): 626.

Morgan, M.K., and Irby, D.M., eds. *Evaluating Clinical Competence in the Health Profession.* St. Louis: C.V. Mosby Co., 1978.

Printen, K.H.; Chapell, W.; and Whitney, D.R. "Clinical Performance Evaluation of Junior Medical Students." *Journal of Medical Education* 48 (1973): 343.

Quarrick, E.A., and Sloop, E.W. "A Method for Identifying the Criteria of Good Performance in a Medical Clerkship Program." *Journal of Medical Education* 47 (1972): 188.

Schwartz, G.F., and Fonnella, J.S. "Measurement of Clinical Competence in the Surgical Clerkship." *Journal of Medical Education* 48 (1973): 762.

Smith, D.L. "Teaching Communications in the Clinical Area." *American Journal of Pharmaceutical Education,* May 1974, p. 186.

Snodgrass, G.L. "Development of a Theoretical Model for Evaluation of Clerkship Experience of Undergraduate Pharmacy Students, thesis. University of Illinois Center for Educational Development, 1977.

Snodgrass, G.L., and Moleski, R.J. "The Process Approach to Clinical Pharmacy Orientation. *American Journal of Hospital Pharmacy* 43 (1979): 142.

Turner, E.V., et al. "Evaluating Clinical Skills of Students in Pediatrics." *Journal of Medical Education* 47 (1972): 959.

Chapter 13

Risk Management

13

No matter what happens, there's always somebody who knew it would.
—Lonny Starr

Many of the functions currently conducted under the auspices of the QA coordinator in hospitals were previously monitored by the risk manager. In many hospitals, risk management predated, and has been integrated into, the newly developed QA program.

Risk management has been defined as loss prevention or liability control. Its purpose is "to eliminate problems that may result in harm to the organization, its staff, and most important, its public."[1] Risk management can also be viewed as a method for improving and maintaining the quality of patient care.[2]

Brown summarizes the basic functions of hospital risk management as follows:[3]

- prevention activities: promoting quality services
- correction activities: rectifying current problems and identifying potential problems
- documentation: keeping records for health, safety, maintenance, and legal functions
- education: training hospital staff and patients
- administration: acting as a staff resource, coordinating existing risk management activities, and implementing needed programs
- environmental control, energy conservation, and infection control.

Some hospitals have designated an individual to coordinate all risk management activities. In other institutions the responsibility for risk management may be delegated to several individuals. The outcome of risk management operations is reported to a safety committee, a QA committee, hospital administration, or any other logical data-collecting body. Regardless of who carries out the functions, certain areas of responsibility are assigned to this component of management. The duties of the risk manager are:[4]

- to develop a system for keeping track of all hospital incidents
- to be responsible for compliance with worker's compensation, Occupational Safety and Health Administration (OSHA), and other applicable regulations
- to act as a member or chairman of safety committee
- to be responsible for security and safety personnel (includes hiring, training)
- to coordinate fire and disaster drills
- to maintain control of keys
- to establish policy and procedure manual to cover such areas as safety, security, and loss prevention
- to conduct hospital inspection tours and security audits
- to periodically review hospital forms used for consent and release activities
- to handle claims filed against the hospital
- to review incident reports
- to participate in hospital quality assurance as related to risk management.

Lenhard referred to risk management with this statement: "Not only should the program be obvious throughout the hospital, but it must be able to be measured."[5] The mutually shared concept of monitoring performance demonstrates one of the relationships between quality assurance and risk management. Other similarities and differences will now be explored in more detail.

To highlight the main difference between these two related disciplines, it might be helpful to remember the analogy of the optimist, who sees the doughnut, and the pessimist, who sees the hole. One's perception depends upon one's point of view. In differentiating quality assurance and risk management, it is essential to focus on the emphasis of the definitions, that is, quality assurance stresses elimination of *problems* that interfere with *quality* of care, while risk management strives to eliminate *risks* that have a potential for financial *loss*.[6] The two approaches to health care management are simultaneously compatible and complementary.

Closer observation reveals that both concepts use the same methodology: identify problems, find causes, take corrective action, assess changes in performance, and so on. Each is also concerned with reducing liability exposure for the institution.

As the national "yardstick" against which hospital care is measured, the Joint Commission on Accreditation of Hospitals (JCAH) standards have begun to stimulate development of hospital-wide QA programs in the United States. Compliance to these guidelines has been established in court as the acceptable level of service to be rendered. Since the establishment of this legal precedent, hospitals have begun to include quality assurance as a necessary component in the overall risk management plan.[7]

The prevention aspect of risk management is explained by Brown in his discussion of the "weed theory of problems."[8] Most problems in the hospital are not solved; they are cut back or mowed down, only to reappear later. Brown maintains that problems can only be eradicated if the roots are destroyed. However, it is not possible to determine whether the roots are really dead until some time has elapsed. Therefore, monitoring of daily incidents becomes necessary.

A "laundry list" of components for QA monitoring of the risk management activities in a hospital (or a department such as pharmacy) is provided below. Using the methodology explained earlier, the manager can develop and implement an effective system for reducing risk and improving patient care. Suggested components in a QA program for risk management include the following:

- complete, comprehensive, and current policies and procedures
- mechanism for tracking all incidents
- ability to recognize problems (e.g., equipment malfunctions, patient falls)
- scheduled inspections for potential hospital safety, fire, and other liability risks
- mechanism for relating QA and risk management activities and eliminating duplication of efforts
- educational programs with documentation
- department checklists to ensure that QA and risk management assessments are conducted and reported as scheduled
- preparation of summaries and reporting of findings to appropriate individuals or committee(s)
- review, at least annually, of complete risk management and QA programs, with documentation
- accountability for ensuring that corrective actions are carried out.

Another example of the overlap of these two activities is shown in Figure 13-1. The dual assessment of health care performance is illustrated in the figure by the shaded areas measured by both quality assurance and risk management. Monagle ties the two concepts together by stating, "As the risk management component of quality assurance improves, patient care will improve, and the first concern of the hospital, the *patient,* will be treated as a whole, human person."[9]

Figure 13-1 Overlap of Risk Management and Quality Assurance in the Assessment of Health Care Performance

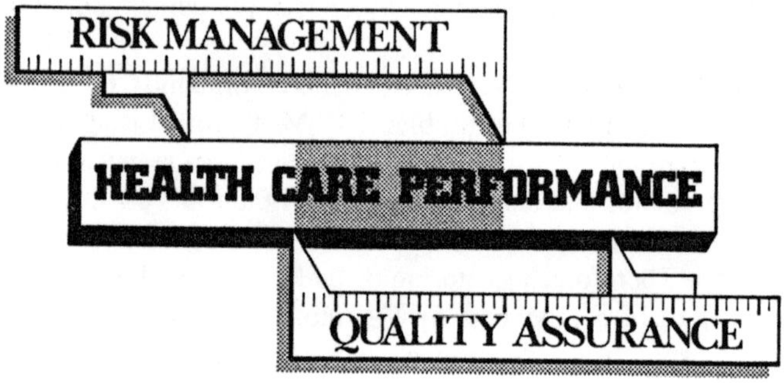

IMPACT OF RISK MANAGEMENT PROGRAMS

One of the dramatic events that established precedents and shaped trends in malpractice claims was the Darling case.[10] Dorrence K. Darling II broke his leg while playing in a football game in 1960. His leg was set at Charleston Community Memorial Hospital. After casting, Darling experienced pain and his toes swelled and became discolored. Eventually Darling's leg was amputated below the knee as a result of impaired circulation in the limb. The patient's father sued the hospital and the physician. The JCAH standards were used as legal evidence for the first time, establishing a precedent for the future. The court ruled in favor of Darling, through two appeals, up to the Illinois Supreme Court. The court held that medical staff bylaws, JCAH regulations, and state licensing requirements could be used as evidence by custom in a malpractice suit, thus effectively establishing an expected level of medical care.[11]

A review of the dramatic increase in malpractice insurance rates in the past decade reflects the awareness of the "expected level of care." For example, malpractice insurance premiums in one hospital rose from $.79 per patient day in 1974 to $11.20 per patient day in 1977. This represents 5 percent of the total cost of caring for the patient.[12] It can be speculated that some of the causes of this increase are higher settlements for suits, patients more willing to sue than in the past, loss of charitable and government immunity by hospitals, and predictions that costs of living and inflation will continue to rise.

The American Hospital Association (AHA) views risk management as the key to prevention of malpractice, by reducing risks to patients in institutions. For progress to occur, the Association also strongly suggests that a long-standing employee attitude must be changed: the former reluctance to "get involved" must be transformed into willingness to report incidents for the benefit of everyone in the hospital.[13]

Brown suggests one method that can create a positive atmosphere among hospital personnel and encourage the "get involved" attitude. When an employee's performance is complimented by a patient, the administrator can commend the employee in a personal note for the individual's demonstration of the hospital's ideals. The public relations value of this gesture can be far reaching and can also be used by any manager in any department of the institution.[14]

ONE AREA TO MONITOR: DRUG ERRORS

In 1978, the Public Health Service and Health Care Financing Administration published a study on medical malpractice claims.[15] The results revealed that 10 percent of the medical malpractice claims reviewed were attributed to drug-related errors.

There are two basic types of drug-related malpractice suits: (1) those attributed to error in dispensing or administering medications and (2) those attributed to drug defects. Of the liability claims involving drugs, one insurance company reported that 74 percent of such claims were due to errors in dispensing, and 22 percent were due to product defects.[16] Therefore, the pharmacist plays a dual role in protecting the patient from hazards of medications. Although the amount of such claims to date has been relatively low (averaging less than $5,000), the number of such claims has increased in the past ten years.[17]

More recently, Steel and associates, in a study of 815 patients on two medical units in a university hospital, revealed that 208 patients developed drug-related complications during their hospital stays.[18] Of all patient complications observed, 53 percent of the patients had at least one problem related to drug exposure. The authors found a positive correlation between drug exposure and development of complications. To bear this out, those patients with no complications received fewer drugs, as compared with the number prescribed for patients receiving medications before the onset of complications developed. The authors established a need to observe patients more closely, stating that "mechanisms must be developed to assess the hazards of hospitalization in an ongoing manner."

Commenting in an editorial on the same subject, Myers suggested that computers be used to record medical data for storage, retrieval, and analysis by physicians.[19] Myers would like to see a national organization, such as the AHA, establish guidelines for monitoring patients. Since 13 percent of hospitalized patients with complex illnesses use 50 percent of a hospital's facilities, the impact of such services is dramatic.

Zellmer points out that neither of these authors recognized that the hospital pharmacist is qualified to conduct drug monitoring services and has already begun to do so in many institutions.[20] This function is a natural outgrowth of the "drug use control" activity of the pharmacist. It seems logical, then, to delegate monitoring of iatrogenic illness to pharmacy. QA audits can easily include criteria for detection of such occurrences. The hospital pharmacist must convince the Pharmacy and Therapeutics Committee and medical staff that monitoring of this type is within the scope of the pharmacist's professional abilities.

Long and Johnson published a hospital incident study to which 18 Iowa hospitals contributed data.[21] Their findings at the end of 1979 showed that 38 percent of the incident reports (the largest category of incidents) were medication errors. This led to a risk management analysis in one participating hospital. The highest risk time periods, patient population, and nursing staff members were identified. Problem causes were recognized and corrective actions were implemented. Medication errors can be reduced, using methods demonstrated in this study, when risk management and quality assurance work together.

CLINICAL PHARMACY AND MALPRACTICE

With the development of clinical pharmacy services, pharmacists are looking forward to playing a more active role in the patient's therapy. Concern has been expressed, however, regarding the liability carried by the pharmacist providing clinical services.

Pharmacists are cautioned that they may be measured against the *physician's* "standard of due care" when consulting and recommending therapy to a physician.[22] Therefore, if a pharmacist provides inaccurate or potentially dangerous information to another health professional, that pharmacist is liable for any harm to the patient that results. In addition, if the professional receiving the information should have recognized that it was wrong, he or she is also liable. Clearly, then, safety mechanisms, in the form of risk management and QA monitoring, must be built into the clinical program to protect the patient's safety. Questions such as, "Was there an unreasonable delay by the pharmacy in providing requested information?" or "Did the pharmacy initiate contact with the physician if potential harm was detected if orders were filled as written?" can be used to measure the effectiveness and safety of services being rendered.[23]

It is also advisable to verify the role that the pharmacist may legally play. In California the pharmacist is permitted to take an active role in assessment of patient needs, while in Ohio a pharmacist providing information on drug therapy would be in violation of the law.[24] This is another example in which knowledge of laws and regulations can reduce liability risks. In addition, pharmacists' performance standards have been established by legal precedent. Two of these measures are (1) degree of skill and care ordinarily possessed by others in the profession and (2) professional standards of practice voluntarily accepted by other members of the profession.[25]

It follows, then, that the pharmacist's responsibilities include monitoring physician's orders for rational therapy and prevention of harm. These functions are usually part of the basic drug distribution and intravenous admixture system in the hospital. Comparison of the results to preestablished QA standards will ensure that these vital functions are performed with the usual degree of skill and care.

COMPENSABLE EVENTS

To broaden the focus from pharmacy-based liability to hospital-wide risk management, problem identification sources will now be examined. Any event resulting in harm to a patient is one in which the hospital may be liable for payment of damages (i.e., a compensable event).

In Virginia hospitals, incident reports have become part of a comprehensive risk management program for identifying patient care problems.[26] This system also compares an individual hospital's incidence of events with comprehensive statewide data to provide a realistic picture of any hospital's actual rate of risk. The next step is the development of corrective actions, tailored to the specific problems being identified. To obtain comparisons on a national level, the reader is referred to the aforementioned (note 15) study conducted by the Department of Health, Education and Welfare in 1978.

By reviewing compensable events, Davis and Bader observed that most medical malpractice claims are both predictable and preventable.[27] They found that a compensable event often follows a series of like events. A pattern of incidents signals a need for corrective action. Therefore, if concurrent monitoring is in effect, it should be possible to detect patterns and prevent further incidents.

For example, if the fact that patients fall out of bed seems to be related to the administration of the patient's hypnotic medications, further investigation is warranted. Physician and nursing education, pertaining to this hazard, would be justified. Careful attention to the use of bed rails must become a standard procedure. Continued monitoring will reveal whether the problem is solved or whether further preventive action is required.

The example cited above illustrates the key to success for risk management or quality assurance: those responsible for patient safety must have the authority to provide prompt action to correct a potential hazard. In addition, medical staff input is required for the planning of corrective action. Without it, cooperation cannot occur.

All health care personnel must remember that "an unhappy patient seems more likely to sue than a satisfied one."[28] One method often used to obtain patient grievance is the use of a patient representative, or ombudsman. This individual is responsible for collecting patient-related problems. Using these data, patterns of behavior can be identified and addressed *before* an incident occurs to harm a patient. The pharmacist often has this same opportunity when he or she is on a nursing unit interacting with patients and medical and nursing personnel. Skillful intervention by a hospital employee can often avoid legal action.

BENEFITS OF HAVING QA PROGRAMS FOR RISK MANAGEMENT

The benefits of a risk management program and a QA program are essentially the same. Some are tangible, others are intangible, but all are valid and demonstrable. By adding quality assurance to the risk management system, the hospital can achieve the benefits of both.

By reducing hazards to the patient, the hospital will develop a reputation for caring about, as well as caring for, the patient. Such an image will encourage physicians and patients to use the services of the hospital more readily. Continued assurance of compliance to safety and accreditation standards can be achieved in an ongoing manner. Management can become proactive instead of reactive, creating a safe and secure environment for patients and employees alike. Post defines a successful risk management program as one that "not only provides an excellent monitor of care but can also alter an existing care system to protect the patient from harm, all in a manner that is cost effective."[29]

As previously mentioned, conducting risk management activities improves communications on all levels in the hospital. Employees are not afraid to "get involved" and to report potentially dangerous situations. Patients' needs are also recognized and answered in a timely manner. Management remains fully informed and, in turn, can then keep employees abreast of developments and plans.

Lastly, a real savings in liability insurance premiums can be demonstrated. The Pennsylvania Insurance Company reported a 9 percent reduction in premiums to member hospitals in 1978 because of risk management efforts.[30] In these times of cost containment and inflation, this last benefit is one that cannot be ignored.

Fink predicts that the trend of the future will take pharmacists in more clinical directions.[31] This transition will require the professional to perform at a higher level than ever before. Legal precedents are leading the patients to expect *maximum* protection from harm. The challenge to health care professionals will continue to grow as the consumer becomes more aware of his or her rights. Quality assurance and risk management are two of the tools available to meet this far-reaching need.

NOTES

1. Bernard L. Brown, Jr., *Risk Management for Hospitals—A Practical Approach* (Rockville, Md.: Aspen Systems Corp., 1979), p. 1.

2. Ibid., p. 2.

3. Ibid., pp. 56-57, 132-133.

4. Ibid., pp. 53-54.

5. Charles G. Lenhard, "Building a Results-Oriented Control Program," *Risk Management*, July 1977, p. 18.

6. John F. Monagle, "The Integration of Risk Management into the JCAH QA Standard," Patient Care Assessment Council Seminar, Orange, California, June 6, 1981.

7. Joseph L. Fink III, "Role of JCAH Standards in Negligence Suits," *American Journal of Hospital Pharmacy* 38 (1981): 892-896.

8. Brown, *Risk Management for Hospitals*, p. 32.

9. John F. Monagle, "Risk Management Is Linked with Quality of Care," *Hospitals* 54, no. 17 (1980): 57-59.

10. Fink, "Role of JCAH Standards in Negligence Suits," p. 893.

11. Joseph L. Fink III, "Some Legal Issues Presented in Clinical Pharmacy Practice," *Drug Intelligence and Clinical Pharmacy* 10 (1976): 444-447.

12. Brown, *Risk Management for Hospitals*, p. 5.

13. Ibid., pp. 10 and 26.

14. Ibid., pp. 17-18.

15. James K. Cooper, ed., "Medical Malpractice Claims: A Synopsis of the HEW/Industry Study of Medical Malpractice Insurance Claims," U.S. Department of Health, Education and Welfare, Public Health Service and Health Care Financing Administration, 1978.

16. Robert S. Beardsley and Albert I. Wertheimer, "Pharmacy Malpractice: Current Status and Trends," *Journal of the American Pharmaceutical Association* 16, no. 10 (1976): 562-564.

17. Ibid.

18. K. Steel et al., "Iatrogenic Illness on a General Medical Service at a University Hospital," *New England Journal of Medicine* 304, no. 11 (1981): 638-642.

19. J.D. Myers, "Preventing Iatrogenic Complications," *New England Journal of Medicine* 304, no. 11 (1981): 664-665.

20. William A. Zellmer, "Can Pharmacists Prevent Drug-Induced Illness in Hospitals?" *American Journal of Hospital Pharmacy* 38, no. 5 (1981): 637.

21. Glenda Long and Colleen Johnson, "A Pilot Study for Reducing Medication Errors," *Quality Review Bulletin*, April 1981, pp. 6-9.

22. Joseph L. Fink III, "Liability of the Pharmacist as a Therapeutic Consultant," *American Journal of Hospital Pharmacy* 38 (1981): 218-222.

23. Ibid.

24. Ibid.

25. Robert F. Steeves and Forrest T. Patterson, "Legal Responsibility of the Hospital Pharmacist for Rational Drug Therapy," *American Journal of Hospital Pharmacy* 26 (1969): 404-407.

26. Richard Oulton, "Use of Incident Report Data in a System-Wide Quality Assurance/Risk Management Program," *Quality Review Bulletin* 7, no. 6 (1981): 2-7.

27. Joseph B. Davis and Barry S. Bader, "The Systems Approach to Patient Safety," *Quality Review Bulletin*, special edition (1979), pp. 79-83.

28. Ruth H. Dudley, "The Patient Representative's Role," *Quality Review Bulletin* 6, no. 4, April 1980, pp. 4-5.

29. Robert S. Post, "Comments on a Pragmatic Route to Quality Assurance," *Quality Review Bulletin* 7, no. 12, December 1981, pp. 4-5.

30. Davis and Bader, "The Systems Approach to Patient Safety," pp. 79-83.

31. Fink, "Some Legal Issues Presented in Clinical Pharmacy Practice," p. 447.

SUGGESTED READINGS

Boxerbaum, Elliott A., and Moore, Timothy D. "Self-Assessment Checklist for Evaluating the Security of a Hospital Pharmacy." *American Journal of Hospital Pharmacy* 38 (1981): 1953-1955.

Brown, Bernard L., Jr. *Risk Management for Hospitals—A Practical Approach*. Rockville, Md.: Aspen Systems Corporation, 1979.

Craddick, Joyce W. "The Medical Management Analysis System." *Quality Review Bulletin*, April 1979, pp. 2-11.

Hoover, Ronald C., et al. "Pilferage of Controlled Substances in Hospital." *American Journal of Hospital Pharmacy* 38 (1981): 1007-1010.

Chapter 14

Drug Utilization Review

14

The art of medicine consists of amusing the patient while nature cures the disease.

—*Voltaire*

The subject of Drug Utilization Review (DUR) as a QA technique was discussed briefly in Chapter 2. In Chapter 3 an explanation of the methodology used to prepare and conduct this type of audit was presented, and in Chapter 13 the concept of the audit process as part of the risk management program in a hospital was developed. In this chapter drug utilization reviews will be examined more intensively, with particular attention to the selection of audit topics and the use of audit results to justify and evaluate pharmaceutical services.

A drug utilization review program has been defined by Stolar as "the system by which quality drug use is defined, measured and ultimately achieved."[1] Drug utilization review techniques are not limited to reviewing prescribing habits of physicians. They can be expanded to encompass other drug-related activities in the pharmacy and multidisciplinary functions throughout the hospital. Examples of other uses of DUR methodology will also be presented in this chapter.

Drug utilization reviews can be used to identify and minimize potential therapeutic problems, such as an inappropriate drug prescribed for intended use, drug overuse, drug underuse, unclear labeling instructions for the patient, potential drug-drug or drug-diet interactions, or potential drug-laboratory test interferences.[2]

Although surveillance of this type has traditionally been used for inpatient monitoring, its use is becoming increasingly recognized for ambulatory patients as well. Palumbo, for example, uses outcome criteria to screen prescriptions for daily dose, quantity prescribed, diagnosis, and labeling information.[3] Ellinoy and co-workers used drug therapy monitoring in an outpatient clinic and listed the following goals for their program:[4]

- to provide continuous, efficient drug utilization reviews
- to promote development of standards for drug therapy
- to identify areas of need for continuing education
- to improve interpersonal relationships
- to improve patient care.

It is vital to develop a climate that will foster the success of the review program. Without an atmosphere of cooperation and trust, the audit activities can easily degenerate into a power struggle or a police action directed against professionals by their peers. In order to establish the required atmosphere, Tremblay suggests several indispensable components:[5]

- objectivity (i.e., the same rules apply to all participants)
- explicit screening criteria developed before beginning data collection
- neutral evaluative position for all participants in the review process (i.e., no power plays are permitted)
- confidentiality of audit findings
- nonthreatening atmosphere (i.e., a positive attitude toward problem solving)
- interpersonal relations based on trust.

Since this atmosphere of trust and confidentiality has been established, it should be possible to extend the use and benefits of DUR methods to many problems in the hospital.

HOW TO SELECT AUDIT TOPICS

Before selecting the specific subject of an audit, it is beneficial to decide on the goal of the review. Retrospective reviews, conducted after patients have been discharged, are easiest to carry out since the patient's medical records are available and usually complete. Results of this type of study cannot help the patients being reviewed but can affect care given to future patients.

Concurrent review has the greatest impact on patients currently in the hospital but may be difficult if all data are not present in the charts during the collection period. An example of an effective program of this type is the review developed by the California Medical Insurance Feasibility Study.[6] It monitors inpatients' records for adverse effects and compares the findings with preestablished criteria. Charts are flagged for immediate follow-up, thereby ensuring that there is an investigation of the situation while the patient is still in the hospital. For such reviews to be effective, however, corrective action must be implemented as soon as the cause of the problem has been identified.[7] In addition to the medical record, there are many other sources that can be used to identify problems in patient care. The reader is referred to Exhibit 2-1 in Chapter 2 for a list of other sources.

Another successful technique for problem identification has been described by Ellinoy as a master problem list.[8] This system uses a permanently numbered, patient-specific list of problems related to health care. It can include information such as diagnosis, unexplained symptoms, physical findings, and laboratory data. The list, if kept current, provides a rapid overview of the total health care situation, highlighting inappropriate or inadequate care. The plan for handling each problem is also recorded. The reference to the medical record makes it possible to track all the events involved in correcting the situation.

Hoffman suggests that the selection of audit topics be based on such factors as the potential for adverse reactions or misuse, the utilization rate of specific drugs, and the relative cost.[9] Although these criteria were designed for judging antibiotic audits, they can be applied to other therapeutic classes of drugs as well.

If the pharmacy uses a computer for data collection and analysis, it is possible to identify highly utilized drugs as potential audit subjects. Computerization may also facilitate sharing information with other departments, thus streamlining the detail work required for audits. Surveys can easily be expanded to include other related disciplines involved in provision of patient care.[10]

After a problem list is compiled, it must be prioritized. It is advisable to keep two major concepts in mind during this process: (1) select those topics to audit that have the potential for the most patient benefit and (2) choose those agents with the greatest potential for patient harm if misused (e.g., anticoagulants).

One specialized field of therapy, worthy of mention as an audit topic, is that of oncology. Agents used to treat neoplastic diseases have potential both for harm and benefit to the patient. Noble and Willoughby suggest four reasons for auditing chemotherapeutic agents:[11]

1. improvement in patient care rendered
2. decrease in hospital liability risks
3. provision of safe working environment for those handling the drugs
4. reduction of hospital and patient care costs due to accurate dosage and fewer side effects.

The subject of chemotherapy provides an opportunity for an audit involving all the disciplines that care for these patients (e.g., physicians, nurses, and pharmacists). The audit criteria should be developed by those practitioners who provide the services being reviewed.

Current therapy of cancer utilizes potent drugs earlier in the treatment and in higher dosages than in the past, which leads to an increased incidence of side effects. Concurrent use of multiple drugs also increases the potential for serious complications. Noble and Willoughby state that "careful monitoring of the patient by the physician, nurse and pharmacist can prevent many of the complications from occurring, or minimizing their effects if they develop."[12]

The following are examples of items that can be included in an audit of oncology drugs:[13]

- Use of warning labels on drug containers prepared in pharmacy such as "Protect from Light" or "Avoid Extravasation."
- placement and size of intravenous catheter
- treatment of extravasation, if it occurs
- use of drug antidotes, when applicable
- disposal of containers and intravenous tubing in contact with an oncology drug.

For an excellent example of an audit on a specific cancer drug, doxorubicin, the reader is referred to the article mentioned in note 11. Other articles describing the hazards of handling antineoplastic agents are listed in the suggested readings at the end of this chapter.

CRITERIA DEVELOPMENT

When writing the criteria against which performance will be measured, it is important to have those who render care involved in the development process. It is also necessary to have the medical staff accept and approve the criteria *before* the data collection phase begins. If the medical staff does not approve the standards, there can be no expectation that the results of the study will be accepted. It follows that corrective action cannot take place if the existence of a problem has not been acknowledged.[14]

Results of an audit must be valid and reliable.[15] Therefore, audit criteria must also be valid, objective, precise, and written in a manner that measures optimum achievable patient care.[16] (A standard is valid if it actually measures what it is supposed to measure.) Brandon and associates suggest that some practical uses of criteria be kept in mind when developing and planning an audit. For example, applying the criteria of an audit to formulary drugs can facilitate medical staff decisions regarding acceptance or deletion of each medication.[17] The authors also suggest that improvements can be encouraged in prescribing habits, if a review is conducted on the directions to the patient typed on prescription labels.[18] Such instructions as "take as directed" are not specific enough to meet established standards.

Stolar proposes that a concurrent audit can be built into a unit dose dispensing system so that all antibiotic orders are automatically screened against previously accepted criteria. The system should be designed to require intervention by the pharmacist if the physician's orders are not in agreement with the established standards.[19]

According to Keyes, the results of an audit must be reliable, that is, if two people use the same set of criteria, their results should be both accurate and consistent. Therefore, audits should include an explanation of any ambiguous terms, numerical values, and sources of information used.[20] Keyes also recommends that no more than ten criteria be used on a review, preferably limiting the list to five or six.

Examples of several specific, measurable audit criteria for a fictitious antibiotic, "Wondermycin," are illustrated in Table 14-1.

Table 14-1 Sample Drug Utilization Review Audit Format for "Wondermycin"

CRITERIA	IDEAL STANDARD	ACTUAL % FOUND	EXCEPTION	DATA SOURCE
1. Patient Parameters				
Age	100%		None	Patient admission info.
Weight (actual)	100%		None	Patient admission info.
Height	100%		None	Patient admission info.
Sex	100%		None	Patient admission info.
History of smoking	100%		None	Patient admission info.
2. Total daily initial dosage not to exceed 5mg/kg/day	100%		None	Physician's order sheet in chart
3. Serum creatinine is drawn within 24 hours of the initiation of therapy.	100%		None	Lab reports in chart
4. Subsequently, serum creatinine is drawn at least every 3 days.	100%		None	Lab reports in chart

Source: Adapted from *Audit Criteria for Aminoglycoside Monitoring,* © 1981. Reprinted with permission by HPI Hospital Pharmacies, Inc.

Once criteria have been established and approved by appropriate individuals, they can be grouped to facilitate the audit process. "Criteria mapping" permits criteria to be grouped according to objectives for the care being rendered.[21] For example, items related to diagnosis of a specific disease would be placed in the same category. The value of the classification of criteria in this manner is that it presents a systematic approach to data collection and display. Logical medical decision making based on audit results is then more likely to occur.

CORRECTIVE ACTIONS

The general subject of corrective actions was presented in Chapter 4. The same remedial principles apply to solving any hospital problem, whether or not it is drug related. The following comments refer to follow-up after drug audits, but the concepts can be applied to improving any situation identified by the QA process.

In institutional health care, there are two basic types of corrective actions, educational and regulatory.[22] Educational programs should stress both the positive and negative aspects of the audit results. Efforts should be made to implement educational efforts that meet the needs of those receiving the information in a timely manner. Programs of this type may be presented in various ways (e.g., formal presentations at medical staff meetings, industry-sponsored continuing education programs, and newsletters). It has been suggested that the best acceptance of educational efforts can be expected when "disease focused" material is presented to physicians and "drug focused" information is given to pharmacists.[23]

Regulatory efforts include such actions as instituting medical staff sanctions regulating privileges and limiting ability to prescribe specific therapeutic agents for the general patient population. Antibiotics often fall into this latter class of drugs. Some hospitals provide special prescription blanks to be used when a "restricted" drug is required. Written documentation justifying the need for the medication and consultation with the infectious disease specialists may also be required before the drug can be administered. In general, regulatory efforts have been found to be more effective than educational programs in affecting prescribing habits of physicians.[24]

Very valid and measurable results can be demonstrated when audits are applied to management of the hospital formulary. Blaufuss indicates that the drug utilization review process, formulary restrictions, and pharmacists monitoring antibiotic dosing are all interrelated programs.[25] Some examples of formulary cost containment achieved through the DUR efforts at St. Elizabeth Hospital in Danville, Illinois are shown in Table 14-2. In addition, the pharmacy at St. Elizabeth Hospital achieved a simultaneous increase in injectable cephalosporin usage, with a projected annual saving for this category of antibiotics of $23,500.

An active QA program that includes drug use review can achieve benefits for the patients and medical staff, as well as for the hospital in general.

Table 14-2 Cost Containment through Formulary Management

<table>
<tr><th></th><th>TYPE OF DRUG</th><th># OF Rx's BEFORE REVIEW</th><th># OF Rx's AFTER REVIEW</th><th>IMMEDIATE SAVING</th><th>ANNUAL SAVING</th></tr>
<tr><td>1.</td><td>Antacids</td><td>14</td><td>3</td><td>$240</td><td rowspan="2">$2,700</td></tr>
<tr><td>2.</td><td>Vitamin-minerals</td><td>57</td><td>20</td><td>$300</td></tr>
<tr><td>3.</td><td>Topical Corticosteroids</td><td>52</td><td>7</td><td>$450</td><td>* N/A</td></tr>
<tr><td>4.</td><td>Cough preps</td><td>37</td><td>11</td><td>$321.70</td><td>* N/A</td></tr>
</table>

* Data for Annual Savings not available

Source: Adapted from John C. Blaufuss, "Cost Containment Through Active Drug-Use Review," *Topics in Hospital Pharmacy Management* 1, no. 3 (1981): 45-52. Reprinted with permission.

REAUDITS

There are several reasons to conduct reaudits. First, reauditing provides a mechanism for determining whether the problem has really been solved. Second, use of the same criteria validates the results of the first audit. Third, as time passes, reaudits ensure that the problem remains corrected. For a detailed discussion of "what to do if the problem isn't solved," the reader is referred to Chapter 4.

When designing an audit, it is important to remember to establish the intervals for reaudits to occur. For example, Baptist Hospital in San Antonio, Texas, conducts two retrospective audits per year on each medical staff problem area. Each hospital department also conducts a concurrent audit on identified problems. Follow-up audits are scheduled every six months.[26]

CONCLUSION

Examples of successful audit programs have been presented with a focus on corrective actions and a discussion of criteria setting. Drug utilization reviews are quality assurance in microcosm, that is, the same terminology and methodology apply to both activities. As such, these reviews should be referred to appropriate hospital committees for review and recommendation. Audits can be conducted manually or with the aid of a computer and can examine the whole spectrum of pharmacologic agents in use in our hospitals. Implementation of the audit process can help:

- to determine whether treatment protocols are effective
- to provide problem identification mechanisms
- to ensure provision of safe and effective therapy
- to reduce health care costs by eliminating duplications of drugs in the formulary.

NOTES

1. Michael H. Stolar, *Psychotropic Drugs—Approaches to Psychopharmacologic Drug Use* (Washington, D.C.: U.S. Government Printing Office, 1979), publication no. 017-024-00926-1, p. 6.
2. Francis B. Palumbo et al., "Detecting Prescribing Problems Through Drug Usage Review: A Case Study," *American Journal of Hospital Pharmacy* 34 (1977): 152-154.
3. Ibid.
4. Brian J. Ellinoy et al., "Pharmacy Audit of Patient Health Records—Feasibility and Usefulness of a Drug Surveillance System," *American Journal of Hospital Pharmacy* 29 (1972): 749-754.
5. Jacques Tremblay, "Creating an Appropriate Climate for Drug Use Review," *American Journal of Hospital Pharmacy* 38 (1981): 212-215.
6. Philip W. Keyes, "Managing an Antibiotic Surveillance Program: Written Criteria and Data Collection," *Current Concepts in Hospital Pharmacy Management*, Fall 1981, pp. 14-18.
7. Ibid.
8. Ellinoy, "Pharmacy Audit of Patient Health Records," pp. 749-754.
9. Richard P. Hoffman, "General Suggestions for Auditing Antibiotic Usage," *Hospital Pharmacy* 15, no. 3 (1980): 143-147.
10. James E. Knoben, "Drug Utilization Review—Current Status and Relationship to Assuring Quality Medical Care," *Drug Intelligence and Clinical Pharmacy* 10 (1976): 222-228.
11. Susan Noble and Patricia W. Willoughby, "Drug Utilization Review for Oncology Drugs: Background and Issues," *Topics in Hospital Pharmacy Management* 1, no. 3 (1981): 65-79.
12. Ibid.
13. Ibid.
14. Hoffman, "General Suggestions for Auditing Antibiotic Usage," pp. 143-147.
15. Keyes, "Managing an Antibiotic Surveillance Program," pp. 14-18.

16. Edward R. Leist and Diane C. Ford, "Pharmacy Strategies for Antibiotic Review," *Topics in Hospital Pharmacy Management* 1, no. 3 (1981): 53-64.

17. Brenda M. Brandon et al., "Drug Usage Screening Criteria," *American Journal of Hospital Pharmacy* 34 (1977): 146-151.

18. Ibid.

19. Michael H. Stolar, "Model for a Formal Prospective Antibiotic Use Review Program," *American Journal of Hospital Pharmacy* 35 (1978): 809-811.

20. Keyes, "Managing an Antibiotic Surveillance Program," pp. 14-18.

21. Sheldon Greenfield et al., "Peer Review by Criteria Mapping: Criteria for Diabetes Mellitus," in *Quality Assurance in Hospitals,* Nancy O. Graham, ed. (Rockville, Md., Aspen Systems Corp., 1982), pp. 149-165.

22. Hoffman, "General Suggestions for Auditing Antibiotic Usage," pp. 143-147.

23. Leist and Ford, "Pharmacy Strategies for Antibiotic Review," p. 65.

24. Hoffman, "General Suggestions for Auditing Antibiotic Usage," pp. 143-147.

25. John C. Blaufuss, "Cost Containment Through Active Drug-Use Review," *Topics in Hospital Pharmacy Management* 1, no. 3 (1981): 45-52.

26. Donna Jones, ed., *Hospital Peer Review* 6, no. 10 (1981): 121-122.

SUGGESTED READINGS

Antibiotic and Drug Use Monitoring Handbook. Chicago: InterQual, 1980.

Hall, Kathy, et al. "Evaluating the Use of Gentamicin in a Small Private Hospital." *Quality Review Bulletin,* special edition, Summer 1981, pp. 40-43.

Harrison, Bruce R. "Developing Guidelines for Working with Antineoplastic Drugs." *American Journal of Hospital Pharmacy* 38 (1981): 1686-1693.

Hendricks, Jacalyn N. *Audit Criteria for Drug Utilization Review.* Washington, D.C.: American Society of Hospital Pharmacists, 1981.

John, Gerald W., and Spieler, John L. "Drug Utilization Review: A Practical Approach." *Hospital Pharmacy* 16, no. 11 (1981): 578-598.

Leist, Edward R., and Ford, Diane C. "Pharmacy Strategies for Antibiotic Review," *Topics in Hospital Pharmacy Management* 1, no. 3 (1981): 53-64.

Visconti, James A. "Drug Use Review," in *Handbook of Institutional Pharmacy Practice,* Mickey Smith and Thomas Brown, eds. Baltimore: Williams & Wilkins, 1979, pp. 363-374.

Zellmer, William. "Reducing Occupational Exposure to Potential Carcinogens In Hospitals," editorial. *American Journal of Hospital Pharmacy* 38 (1981): 1679.

Zimmerman, Paul F., et al. "Recommendations for the Safe Handling of Injectable Antineoplastic Drug Products." *American Journal of Hospital Pharmacy* 38 (1981): 1693-1695.

Chapter 15

Outpatient Dispensing Activities

15

Usually, the hospital pharmacist's training and work experience are directed primarily toward the nonambulatory inpatients of the institution. Nevertheless, most hospital pharmacies conduct outpatient dispensing activities, to some degree, as part of the dispensing operations. The functions relating to outpatients are often looked upon as a small, required part of the pharmacy, provided merely as a service, with little if any profit to be realized. It is this very opinion that illustrates the need for quality assurance in outpatient dispensing. It is natural for the pharmacist to spend as little time as possible in this area; therefore, controls can easily become lax. The QA program established in the outpatient area can certify that all requirements are met and that all prescriptions are dispensed with 100 percent accuracy. For the purpose of this discussion, outpatients will include the following categories of individuals who may have a prescription filled in the hospital pharmacy:

- Emergency department patients
- Worker's compensation patients
- Clinic patients
- Inpatients taking medications home upon discharge
- Employees of the hospital
- Interns, residents, and students
- Physicians and members of their immediate families.

No "walk in" patients may be included. The reason for this exclusion will be explained in detail later in this chapter.

Palumbo and associates graphically demonstrated the need for some form of monitoring in outpatient drug therapy in a study published in 1977.[1] An audit was conducted of 1,033 prescription orders in an outpatient clinic, which measured four prescribing and dispensing parameters: (1) daily dose prescribed, (2) quantity of drug prescribed and dispensed, (3) diagnosis, and (4) labeling. They found that 574, or 56 percent, failed one or more criteria. The most common failing was found to be prescribed dosages below the accepted minimum range, especially for antibiotics. A total of 4 percent had inadequate labeling of directions for use (e.g., take as directed).

Various professional organizations have also recognized the need for more structure and have recommended guidelines or standards for outpatient dispensing functions. The American Pharmaceutical Association (APhA), for example, published "Standards of Practice for the Profession of Pharmacy" in 1979.[2] These standards detail procedures involved in the correct handling of prescriptions. Section II is recommended as a starting point for development of a QA program for outpatient dispensing. Even the Joint Commission on Accreditation of Hospitals (JCAH) includes a few guidelines pertaining to medications for outpatients, such as those listed below:

- It is the responsibility of the pharmacy staff to establish the identity of the patients, or the person accepting prescription medication for an outpatient. A written procedure should be available to cover this procedure.[3]
- A mechanism should be available for the pharmacist's use, which verifies the name, signature, and Drug Enforcement Agency (DEA) number assigned to each prescriber.[4]

LABELING

One of the most important areas to be reviewed involves the accuracy of the label presented to the patient. The label, which accompanies the medication for the duration of therapy, is the continuing source of information on how to take the drug. Much has been written on the subject of label requirements. To obtain a list of mandatory label components, the federal and state regulations that apply to pharmacy practice in a specific geographical location must be checked.

Zelonis and associates also provided a list of required items for prescription labels.[5] In addition, the JCAH standards provide a similar list, containing a few additional components.[6] A combination of these two lists of suggested elements for outpatient prescription labels is presented below:

- Pharmacy's name, address, and telephone number
- Prescription number
- Patient's name and address
- Directions for use

- Prescriber's name and DEA number (when appropriate)
- Date of issue of prescription
- Initials of pharmacist filling prescription
- Name of drug, strength, and amount dispensed (with prescriber's approval)
- Lot number and expiration date of drug
- Auxiliary labels, when necessary (including DEA caution label)

Once the elements for a label have been established, written, and approved, each person working in the outpatient area should be familiar with the requirements. Sample labels may be posted for reference. Auditing label accuracy can be done randomly, on a preestablished number of prescriptions. The results of this audit comprise one facet of the QA program.

OTHER SUGGESTED SUBJECTS TO BE MONITORED

The correctness and completeness of labels are only two of the elements to be reviewed. A sampling of other topics is presented below, expressed as a list of questions. The reviewer can ask any or all of these questions while surveying outpatient dispensing practices. Negative or incomplete answers will indicate subjects for further study or corrective action.

- Has the prescription been filled with the prescribed drug (or its approved generic equivalent)? Was the correct strength of the drug dispensed?
- Is the amount of the drug dispensed the same as the amount prescribed? Will the quantity be sufficient for the duration of therapy?
- Will the drug have sufficient shelf life to permit usage for the duration of therapy?
- Is the diagnosis of the patient one of the indications for the drug?
- Is the prescribed dosage within the normal range?
- Is the duration of therapy within the usual limits?
- Are there any known drug interactions with other drugs being used concomitantly?
- If patient profiles are in use in the outpatient area, are drug allergies, diagnosis, patient weight, and age recorded on the profile?
- How many refills have been authorized? How many have been used? Are they recorded as required by law?
- Was the correct type of prescription container used for the drug? Was a waiver signed if a non-child-proof container was dispensed?

- Does the patient's address appear on controlled drug prescriptions? Is the prescriber's DEA number also present?
- Was the patient counseled or given appropriate patient package inserts, as required? Was the counseling documented?
- Are the lot number, manufacturer, and expiration date of the drug dispensed written on the prescription? In the event of a recall is there a way to contact the patient if necessary?
- Is the price charged the patient within the pharmacy or hospital price guidelines?
- Was the length of time required for the patient to wait for the prescription within acceptable, predetermined limits?
- How often is the prescribed drug out of stock? Is permission obtained to use an alternative drug, when appropriate? How long is the delay before the prescription can be filled?
- Are separate files maintained for controlled drug prescriptions, as required?
- Are retail permits or licenses on display, as required?

CONTROLLED SUBSTANCE PROCEDURES

The special procedures that are required for outpatient controlled drug prescriptions and files are similar to those used for inpatient records. If there is a large outpatient prescription volume, separate stocks of controlled substances may be warranted, with their respective records and files. Separate inventories may be required anyway, since most inpatient stock will probably be in unit dose form, which is not easily or quickly adapted to outpatient dispensing.

When the biannual controlled substance inventory is taken in May of every odd-numbered year, the outpatient stock must also be included. Review of stock for expired and recalled drugs must encompass outpatient inventory as well.

Separate prescription files for Schedule II drugs should be maintained. DEA regulations also specify a file for invoices of Schedule II drugs. All of the regulations pertaining to management and record keeping for controlled substances mentioned previously also apply in the outpatient area. Review of perpetual inventory records should also show deductions of quantities used for outpatient prescriptions.

If state law requires specific information to be recorded on the prescription blank, for copies of multipart forms to be mailed in, or for a monthly summary of Schedule II drugs to be performed, then these copies and reports should also be reviewed as a regular part of the QA program.

Poison or exempt narcotic registers are required in some states. This is one point to verify in the state and local pharmacy regulations and to include in the QA section for outpatient dispensing, if necessary.

USE OF ANCILLARY PERSONNEL

Hospital pharmacies traditionally employ technicians, students, and interns to assist with routine tasks. Most state laws are specific with regard to which functions *must* be performed by a pharmacist and which ones *may* be done by nonlicensed personnel under a pharmacist's supervision. After reviewing the law, one may ask several questions pertaining to such functions. For example:

- Who may take a prescription over the telephone?
- Who may accept authorization for a refill over the telephone?
- How are refill authorizations verified and documented?
- Are there limitations on who may select the drug, "count or pour," type, or affix the label?
- What final checks are built into the dispensing system?
- Who may hand the prescription container to the patient?
- Is there a ratio specified in the law concerning how many ancillary personnel one pharmacist may supervise? Has this ratio been followed or exceeded?

SEPARATE INVENTORY REQUIREMENTS

At the beginning of this chapter, specific categories of patients were defined under the umbrella term *outpatient*. If prescriptions are filled in a hospital pharmacy for patients in any other category, the pharmacy is then considered to be in competition with retail establishments. Therefore, drugs purchased from suppliers using hospital discounts and bids must not be used for outpatient prescriptions. Separate outpatient inventories will be required, purchased at prices competitive with those paid by retail establishments. To reiterate, this separation of inventories is *not* required when outpatients can be classified in one of the following categories:[7]

- inpatients still in the hospital
- patients using medications in the emergency department
- outpatients using medications on hospital premises

- inpatients or emergency department patients using medication after discharge, away from hospital premises
- outpatients using medication away from hospital premises
- hospital employees or students using medications for their own personal use or for use by their dependents
- physicians on the medical staff using medication for personal use or for use by their dependents.

These categories were defined by the U.S. Supreme Court after the Portland Retail Druggist Association sued Abbott Laboratories, and other suppliers, for price discrimination. The association accused the manufacturers of selling products to hospital pharmacies at prices lower than those charged retail establishments.

It is prudent for the hospital pharmacist to conduct a careful review of the types of patients having prescriptions filled. If categories other than those on the above list are identified, it may be necessary to limit the service or to maintain a separate inventory.

There is another regulation that affects purchases of drugs sold to outpatients: the Robinson-Patman Act, passed in 1936. This act prohibits price discrimination and was the basis of the aforementioned suit against Abbott Laboratories and other suppliers. In 1938, the Non-Profit Institutions Act included hospitals under the exempt institutions protected by this act, as long as the items purchased were being used by the hospitals themselves.[8] If the court rules that a hospital is in violation of the Robinson-Patman Act, penalties could include payments of up to three times the amount of damages suffered by the plaintiff. Violators can also be subject to criminal sanctions.[9]

In light of the legal precedents already established, the QA standards for outpatient dispensing become quite necessary, and also cost effective!

TAKE-HOME MEDICATIONS

There is a certain degree of overlap into other phases of pharmacy operations when one considers prescriptions filled in the hospital pharmacy to be taken home with the patient. For example, the JCAH requires that such medications be appropriately labeled and written into the patient's medical record.[10] The required labeling and charting procedures encompass both inpatient and outpatient activities. The JCAH also specifies that, upon order of a physician, the patient be instructed as to the correct use of the take-home drugs.[11] Obviously, the counseling of the patient is a common area, mutually shared by the outpatient and clinical pharmacy services. Design of the QA program should take these mutual areas into consideration, both to provide complete coverage and to prevent duplication. The topics to be audited for take-home prescriptions include the same areas as for other outpatient medications, with a few exceptions:

- Is the quantity of medication sufficient for the patient's therapy? Are limits placed on the amount of analgesics or hypnotics for the patient's home use?
- Was the patient or a family member counseled regarding safe and correct use of the drugs? Was the counseling process documented?
- Was the prescription sent to the pharmacy with sufficient lead time so that the patient was not kept waiting upon discharge?
- Were the prescriptions recorded on the patient's medical record and the pharmacy medication profile?
- Is the prescription charge to be added to the patient's bill, or does the patient pay for the medication when it is received? Are charges turned in with the patient's discharge billing records to avoid late charges?

HANDLING OF CASH, CHECKS, AND CHARGES

The last point mentioned above leads into the general discussion of controls for cash, checks, and charges. This area is a facet of outpatient procedure that requires specific, written policies for employees to follow. In some hospitals, the pharmacy never handles the payment for the medication (i.e., the patient pays the business office). Pharmacy personnel release the prescription to the patient when a receipt copy is presented. Most hospital pharmacies, however, use more common billing methods, such as adding charges to the inpatient bill for appropriate take-home medications (e.g., in worker's compensation cases) or collecting directly from the patient.

Policies covering the control of money can be used as the basis for checking on the accuracy of the system. The following are some subjects to be included in these policies:

- Who may handle cash?
- What security systems protect the people, drugs, and money in the outpatient area?
- How are shortages and overages handled? How frequently do they occur?
- How frequently are cash deposits made, by whom, and to whom?
- What system is used for obtaining personal identification when accepting payment by check?
- Are prescriptions billed with inpatient charges handled in a timely manner, to avoid late charges?

- What is the minimum amount of money to be kept on hand, in what denominations?
- Is there a policy for handling welfare or other special types of prescriptions? Is it being followed? Is the policy posted prominently in the outpatient area?
- Is there a mechanism for replacing money "paid out" of the cash supply?

DRUG RECALLS

In recent years, JCAH inspectors have become aware of the outpatient phase of hospital pharmacy. They often ask how drug recalls are handled when an outpatient has received a prescription for a recalled drug. The pharmacy must have a mechanism for tracing recalls through outpatient prescriptions and for contacting the patient when necessary. Therefore, lot number, manufacturer, and expiration date information should be recorded on the prescription when it is filled or refilled. It has also been suggested that a means for contacting the physician be established in the event that a drug recall involves a life-threatening situation.[12]

DRUG UTILIZATION REVIEWS AND OTHER PATIENT CARE AUDITS

Ambulatory care patient records provide a fund of information no less important than that provided by inpatient records. The potential for learning from this information source should not be overlooked. Once again, virtually every aspect of patient care offered to inpatients can also be examined in the outpatient setting. It may be necessary to tailor the standards to fit the specific patient needs involved, but the results of all audits should provide equally valuable information. For examples of ambulatory-care patient audits, the reader is referred to the suggested readings at the end of this chapter.

Outpatients have the same right to quality medical care as do inpatients. They deserve the same assurances of safety and accuracy provided for hospitalized patients. If an inpatient develops an adverse effect to a medication, the health care team is ready to provide assistance. Medicating the outpatient, however, is usually out of the span of control of hospital personnel. The instructions given to the outpatient, therefore, become even more important as the patient recuperates at home.

Finally, the usual attitude of most hospital pharmacists is that the outpatient department is a "stepchild," and this opinion emphasizes the need for safeguards. A complete QA program in a hospital pharmacy includes both the outpatient operations and the inpatient functions of the department.

NOTES

1. Frances B. Palumbo et al., "Detecting Prescribing Problems Through Drug Usage Review: A Case Study," *American Journal of Hospital Pharmacy* 34 (1977): 152-154.
2. Samuel H. Kalman and John F. Schlegel, "Standards of Practice for the Profession of Pharmacy," *American Pharmacy* NS19, no. 3 (1979): 21-33.
3. *Accreditation Manual for Hospitals* (Chicago: Joint Commission on Accreditation of Hospitals, 1981), p. 143.
4. Ibid., p. 141.
5. Anthony Zelonis et al., "A Pharmacy Quality Assurance Program," *Hospital Formulary*, February 1979, pp. 205-211.
6. *Accreditation Manual for Hospitals*, p. 143.
7. Michael K. Fire, "Hospital Procurement and Illegal Price Discrimination," *Hospital Materiel Management Quarterly* 1 (1979): 53-59.
8. Ibid.
9. Ibid.
10. *Accreditation Manual for Hospitals*, p. 145.
11. Ibid., p. 142.
12. Charles E. Drake and Hugh F. Kabot, "A Quality Assurance Program for Pharmaceutical Purchases," *Journal of the American Pharmaceutical Association* NS11, no. 11 (1971): 612-615.

SUGGESTED READINGS

Bressler, Linda, et al. "Drug Use Review in Ambulatory Care Centers." *Journal of Ambulatory Care Management*, May 1981, pp. 57-68.

Carpenter, John K. "A Method of Monthly Peer Review for the Emergency Department." *Journal of Ambulatory Care Management*, July 1978, pp. 97-100.

Currey, Clarence, E., et al. "Audit of Phenytoin Prescribing for Outpatients." *American Journal of Hospital Pharmacy* 38 (1981): 1158-1160.

Ellinoy, Brian J., et al. "A Pharmacy Outpatient Monitoring Program Providing Primary Medical Care to Selected Patients." *American Journal of Hospital Pharmacy* 30, no. 7 (1973): 593-598.

Solomon, David, K., et al. "Use of Medication Profiles to Detect Potential Therapeutic Problems in Ambulatory Patients," in *Clinical Pharmacy Sourcebook*, William Zellmer, ed. Washington, D.C.: American Society of Hospital Pharmacists, 1976, pp. 134-140.

Chapter 16

Evaluation and Reassessment of the Pharmacy Department's QA Program

16

History repeats itself. That's one of the things wrong with history.
—Clarence Darrow

In this chapter two related topics will be examined: (1) the evaluation of the QA program and (2) the methods of reassessment that can be used as part of the QA program. Evaluation of the program provides an opportunity to determine whether the goals and objectives of the program are being met. Reassessment is a method used to determine and document the extent of problem resolution. Since problem resolution is one of the fundamental goals of the QA program, the two processes are related.

EVALUATION OF THE QA PROGRAM

Although the JCAH standards relating to quality assurance require at least annual review and evaluation of the program, it may be advisable to conduct the appraisal more frequently during the early phases.[1] Evaluation can provide the following types of information:

- whether the goals and objectives of the program are being met
- whether the strengths of the program are being maintained and the weaknesses corrected
- whether the program is keeping pace with the evolution of new standards and advances in technology.[2]

Kaplan and Hopkins suggest that four main areas be included in the overall appraisal of the QA program. These areas are (1) organization of the program, (2) problem-focused approach, (3) mechanisms for reporting, and (4) impact of the program.[3]

Since the evaluation process is a retrospective review, it is appropriate to focus on the results of the program. It may be helpful to ask any or all of the following questions during the appraisal process:

- Can improvement in patient care be demonstrated?
- Was the effort expended to solve problems cost effective?
- Was a solution found for each problem addressed?
- Is each standard in each area of the QA program still current, or is revision required?

In addition to the use of reassessment, which will be described in greater detail later in the chapter, several other techniques may be of value. For example, surveys may be conducted that ask patients, hospital employees, and the medical staff to evaluate pharmacy services. The results can then be incorporated into the overall evaluation. It is not recommended that the survey results be used as the entire evaluation because the responses will be subjective.

The review of pharmacy services conducted by the pharmacy and therapeutics committee (described in Chapter 11) should also be included in the total appraisal. It also may be advisable to allow an outside observer to conduct an on-site inspection, comparing actual performance against reported compliance to standards. This technique is the one used to validate the QA program in pharmacies managed by HPI Hospital Pharmacies, Inc.[4]

When the evaluation process has been completed, results should be reported to those who have authority over the program (e.g., the QA director, administrator, or director of pharmacy). Care should be taken to maintain confidentiality. If the results of the measurement process reveal the need for changes in the program, then those who have authority over the QA program must be responsible for approving proposed alterations in it.[5] It is recommended that these points of accountability and authority be clearly delineated in the hospital's QA plan.

REASSESSMENT

Reassessment is used to document the extent of problem resolution achieved by the QA program. It is suggested that reassessment be planned and defined when corrective actions are selected. Care must be taken to ensure that the same measurement instrument is used for both the assessment and reassessment phases.

When establishing parameters for the reassessment phase, the planners should consider and determine each of the following components:

- extent of desired problem resolution (or changes) expected
- time frame and date of reassessment
- sample size for reassessment
- responsibility for reassessment process
- methodology for reassessment process[6]
- format for reporting results.

It is possible that the results of reassessment will reveal that a problem has not been solved. A detailed discussion of this contingency is provided in Chapter 4.

Providers of a service that is being evaluated could try to deceive the observer. Suchman has identified two terms used to describe methods for avoiding or preventing perception of reality.[7] They are *eyewash* and *whitewash*. Eyewash is an attempt at making things look better than they are. Whitewash involves covering up unacceptable practices. If the criteria used on assessment and reassessment are written in a measurable style, and the surveys are scrupulous in presenting results, then neither eyewash nor whitewash techniques will be possible.

DEMONSTRATING THE VALUE OF THE QA PROGRAM

After expending the effort to develop, implement, and validate a QA program, the pharmacist should be able to reap the benefits. The overall benefits of the QA program will be discussed in Chapter 18. The following comments will be limited to establishing credibility after the evaluation of the QA program.

One of the most urgent requirements for any program in health care is its cost effectiveness. It should not be difficult to establish measurable benefits of the QA program in the pharmacy. Two areas can easily provide evidence of financial benefits, that of inventory management and Drug Utilization Review (DUR). It has been documented that, when recommendations are followed subsequent to DURs, the incidence of medication side effects may be reduced and the length of stay can be shortened.[8,9] It can also be shown, using the results of reassessment, that pharmacy inventory can be decreased through adherence to bids and other fiscal management techniques.[10,11]

Properly conducted, the QA program can keep the pharmacy in a state of readiness for any inspection. When an inspection is conducted, the pharmacy department can expect, and receive, high marks for compliance to regulations and the presence of an active QA program. Commendations of this type are often sufficient justification for continuation of QA activities.

CONCLUSION

Reporting results of annual reassessment provides the pharmacist with an opportunity to remind the administration and medical staff of the positive achievements of the department. Conducting the annual review also ensures that all previously established controls are still effective. Finally, the reassessment process may identify further problems, new ones, those previously solved, and problems that had been recognized but not solved. Prioritizing new problems along with those already identified provides direction for continuity of QA efforts.

NOTES

1. *Accreditation Manual for Hospitals* (Chicago: Joint Commission on Accreditation of Hospitals, 1981), p. 153.

2. Karen O. Kaplan and Julie M. Hopkins, *The QA Guide—A Resource for Hospital Quality Assurance* (Chicago: Joint Commission on Accreditation of Hospitals, 1980), p. 129.

3. Ibid., pp. 130-131.

4. Kenneth N. Horowitz and Marlene Lamnin, "Design and Implementation of a Quality Assurance Program for Pharmaceutical Services," *American Journal of Hospital Pharmacy* 37 (1980): 82-84.

5. Kaplan and Hopkins, *The QA Guide*, p. 129.

6. Ibid., pp. 125-126.

7. E.A. Suchman, "Action for What? Critique of Evaluation Research," in *Evaluating Action Programs: Readings in Social Action and Education*, C.H. Wiess, ed. (Boston: Allyn & Bacon, 1972), pp. 52-84.

8. Susan Noble and Patricia W. Willoughby, "Drug Utilization Review for Oncology Drugs: Background and Issues," *Topics in Hospital Pharmacy Management* 1, no. 3 (1981): 65-79.

9. John C. Blaufuss, "Cost Containment Through Active Drug-Use Review," *Topics in Hospital Pharmacy Management* 1, no. 3 (1981): 45-52.

10. Jack McPartland, "Alternative Medication for Outpatients Provides Savings," *Hospital Pharmacy* 15 (1980): 424-425.

11. J.V. Anandan, "Reducing the Number of Formulary Theophylline Preparations," *American Journal of Hospital Pharmacy* 38 (1981): 511-513.

Chapter 17

Quality Assurance As a Management Tool

17

When you're thirsty, it's too late to think about digging a well.
—Anonymous

In Chapter 10 the use of QA activities to monitor management functions was discussed. In this chapter the opposite viewpoint will be examined: that the manager can use QA techniques as tools to improve efficiency, ensure compliance to regulations, reduce liability risks, and achieve established goals. The topics within the scope of management discussed in this chapter include personnel activities, fiscal responsibilities, legal mandates, goal development and achievement, and risk reduction.

PERSONNEL ACTIVITIES

The assessment mechanisms that a manager develops to measure performance of personnel can be used to identify the need for training, retraining, or counseling of staff members. Patterns of lateness, chronic absenteeism, types and frequency of drug errors, and other critical factors can be used to identify problems requiring investigation and possible action by the manager. On a more positive note, excellence in performance can also be recognized and rewarded if a system is established to document the presence of compliance to behavioral objectives.

Grogan, in an interview published in *Topics in Hospital Pharmacy Management*, indicated the need for the hospital pharmacist to be aware of the entire hospital's QA plan. Of course, the manager should also be involved in internal quality assurance, ensuring that there are adequate procedures for monitoring work performance and that people are paid according to the quality of their work.[1] According to Grogan, the manager's charge—to assess the quality of work performance—is facilitated by the use of QA techniques.

Furthermore, the manager must be able to detect personnel problems and resolve them as quickly as possible. Employees recognize this ability (or the lack of it) as a key factor in the management style of the supervisor. Golightly summarizes conflict recognition skills as follows, "The manager who understands how conflicts originate and how people deal with them is prepared to confront disruptive situations. Staff members will seek the leadership of a manager who can help them confront conflict as a preliminary step toward problem-solving."[2]

FISCAL RESPONSIBILITIES

From the manager's perspective, financial responsibilities are among the most critical aspects in the job description. Development of a budget conservative enough to be approved, yet liberal enough to permit growth, is an annual challenge. Monthly reports remind the manager of his or her skill in meeting goals, reducing costs, and increasing revenue. The budget monitors described in Chapter 10 assist the manager in detecting problems and in planning for methods to keep financial results within the accepted limits.

Checks on accuracy of patient billing, frequency of lost charges for stock drugs, and incidence of late charges will inform the manager of potential sources of lost revenue. The control of drug charging is related to the accuracy of pricing methods, used when items are purchased and received. The entire realm of inventory control is intimately related to the efficient fiscal operation of the pharmacy department, under the guidance of the manager. All of the monitors established for inventory control and for patient charging will assist the manager in meeting predetermined financial goals. Therefore, it is urgent that QA standards for the aforementioned areas are established, kept current, and assessed frequently.

LEGAL MANDATES

The QA program in the pharmacy can assist the manager in ensuring that licenses are current, records are properly maintained and stored, and all regulatory requirements are completely met. The vast number of legal details can be reduced to simple checklists, which provide systematic techniques for the manager's use. Included in these controls should be guarantees that controlled substances and alcohol are properly secured. Purchasing and dispensing of both substances require very specific records. Again, quality assurance can ensure that stringent controls are exercised and documented. A study by Hoover and associates places responsibility for management of medications in the hospital quite specifically:

"Drug control is a major aspect of the pharmacists' management responsibility."[3] In this study, the authors estimated that 500,000 dosage units, or more, are pilfered in hospitals in the United States per year, especially those drugs having a high abuse potential. They recommend stringent controls and frequent periodic audits. A QA system, covering all aspects of drug dispensing and administration, will help prevent opportunities for pilferage of this type to occur.

The department's policy and procedure manual should meet specific requirements for its contents and receive approval by specified individuals. Once again, QA methodology will facilitate production and maintenance of an informative manual, one that meets both external and internal requirements.

Checks on dispensing for various categories of outpatients are also necessary. Here is one area in which hospital pharmacy interfaces with the life of the patient outside the institution. It is therefore even more important that controls prevent error and assist the patient in the proper use of medications. Patient education programs coupled with cost-effective puchasing are two mechanisms that the pharmacist may use to demonstrate the value of pharmacy's services to the patient. The astute manager recognizes the potential for improving pharmacy's professional image when outpatients are provided with individualized services that meet their specific needs. Necessary documentation maintained in the outpatient area will further ensure compliance to regulations and patient safety.

GOAL DEVELOPMENT AND ACHIEVEMENT

One significant measure of a manager is the achievement of established goals. As we have discussed above, one of the best methods for selection of relevant goals is to review the problems detected by the QA process. Employees usually accept the need for activities that produce an improvement in patient care. Therefore, quality assurance affords the manager the advantage of achieving goals that solve problems, while raising the level of patient care. Moreover, when employees develop pride in obtaining predetermined goals, a positive morale factor has been introduced into the working environment.

Once the corrective action has solved the original problem, the manager reassesses the situation. By this time, several objectives should have been accomplished:

- A patient care problem has been solved.
- The manager's goal has been achieved.
- Employees have been involved in solving problems.
- QA operations have documented the results.

For the planning and achieving of specific management objectives, the health care manager has one of the most versatile instruments at his or her disposal: the QA system.

RISK REDUCTION

Whether or not risk management is handled by a discrete department or an individual in the hospital, risk control is a vital component of the pharmacist's job. Drug error review and prevention is one of the most important responsibilities of every pharmacist. Controls must be built into each facet of pharmacy operations to ensure that safe and effective drugs are dispensed. The "rights" of the patients must be fulfilled: right drug, right dosage, right time, right mode of administration, and right patient.

The pharmacist is also responsible for selection of safe and effective medications obtained from reliable sources. Drug recalls, with appropriate documentation, must be handled carefully. Drug defects must be reported to the Food and Drug Administration and to the manufacturer as soon as they are detected. Moreover, employee health and safety must always be safeguarded. Educational programs provided by the hospital or the pharmacy should cover topics such as fire and accident prevention, infection control, disaster drills, and occupational hazard recognition. Current documentation of employee attendance at educational programs must be maintained. As the discussion in Chapter 13 indicates, risk management and quality assurance are two closely related functions that are opposite but equal in emphasis.

CONCLUSION

The discussion on quality assurance for clinical services in Chapter 12 demonstrated the concept that both professional services and personnel competence can be evaluated using the same basic monitoring techniques. The identical principle can be applied, generally, to evaluations by the manager of personnel and procedures in the pharmacy department. Whether performing an analysis on the impact of services or on the competency of aseptic techniques demonstrated in the intravenous admixture program, the manager can use the same evaluative tools. Because of the adaptability of QA techniques to any situation, health care professionals have endorsed and encouraged their use.

The pharmacist-manager might be compared to an artist standing before a blank canvas. In order to produce the desired painting, the artist may have to use a variety of brushes. Each has its specific function, and each contributes to the completion of the whole creation. If the manager is to integrate all of the functions performed by each employee in the department into one coordinated service unit, he or she must use all the tools available to expedite the task. QA monitors, built into every aspect of both department performance and interprofessional activities, give the manager the full range of "brushes" needed to create a comprehensive composition.

NOTES

1. "Perspectives on Pharmacy and Quality Assurance—A Talk with Jim Grogan," *Topics in Hospital Pharmacy Management* 1, no. 3 (1981): 91-99.

2. Cecilia K. Golightly, *Creative Problem Solving for Health Care Professionals* (Rockville, Md.: Aspen Systems Corp., 1981), p. 21.

3. Ronald C. Hoover et al., "Pilferage of Controlled Substances in Hospitals," *American Journal of Hospital Pharmacy* 38 (1981): 1007-1010.

Chapter 18

Results of a QA Program

18

Quality is never an accident. It is always the result of intelligent effort.
—John Ruskin

Throughout this text there are many references to outcomes and results. What are the results that can be achieved after a QA program has been implemented? Several approaches to finding answers for this question are now presented.

REGULATORY REQUIREMENTS

The first and most obvious answer is that a QA program provides the health care manager with a means to meet all regulatory requirements. Standards—promulgated by the Joint Commission on Accreditation of Hospitals (JCAH), Medicare, federal and state laws, and guidelines from professional organizations—all can be combined in the design of the QA program. In addition, the same standards can be used as a checklist to prepare for audit visits by various inspectors.

Current economic conditions are affecting both governmental and voluntary accrediting organizations. As governmental fiscal constraints reduce funding to health-related agencies, the interval between inspections becomes longer and longer. The JCAH has begun awarding three-year accreditations to hospitals that qualify, while one- and two-year awards are still possible.

A QA program in the pharmacy contributes to the overall compliance of the hospital to regulatory requirements, especially during the period between inspections. Participation and documentation by the pharmacy in the hospital-wide QA plan should be one of the cornerstones upon which the plan is built. In general, QA programs have been described as management systems that use the JCAH's standards as a focal point, from which all other standards emanate.[1]

DEMONSTRATION OF PROFESSIONAL ABILITIES

The problem-identification phase of quality assurance can provide the professional with a rare opportunity to design and monitor new services that will meet the needs of the patients. An article published in a 1978 issue of *Hospitals* described just such an opportunity.[2] A questionnaire was distributed to patients, asking them to evaluate the quality of pharmaceutical services provided at the hospital. The responses of the patients indicated that they recognized the value of counseling, regarding prescription medications, conducted by pharmacists. In fact, patients expressed the desire for available counseling in the community setting as well as in the hospital. An evaluation of this type is vital to those individuals providing the service. Pharmacists participating in the aforementioned counseling service found that the patients' responses helped them whenever necessary to revise the program. Further, the medical staff was pleased with the program and expressed their satisfaction to the pharmacy staff.

Without a method of evaluating the quality of a service, how can the impact of the service be determined? How can the need for modification of the service or training of staff members be established? Without quality assurance, pharmacists have a case of never knowing whether the destination has been reached, because they cannot measure how far, or in what direction, they have traveled.

Establishment of a service tailored to solve a problem or fulfill a need represents an opportunity to translate theory into action. The professional can demonstrate the knowledge and willingness needed to implement the required program. Once reassessment of the situation documents that the problem is solved, the QA cycle is complete.

Implementation of new services may also be an opportunity to generate additional revenue for the department. Identification of potential new revenue sources is a challenge faced by all health care managers, regardless of background or training. Quality assurance can give the manager a road map leading in the direction of potential new funding methods.

WORKING WITH OTHER PROFESSIONALS

The multidisciplinary characteristics of the JCAH standard for quality assurance have given the pharmacist the chance to work with others in the health care institution. To look at it another way, working with other professionals places the pharmacist in a position to participate in QA functions of a multidisciplinary nature. Involvement in such routine events as committee meetings, physicians' rounds, clinical services, pharmacy-based intravenous therapy, and home health care should help to establish the pharmacist as an integral member of the team to provide and evaluate patient services. Moreover, participation of this nature will enhance the pharmacist's credibility among other health care providers.

DOCUMENTING IMPROVEMENT IN PHARMACY DEPARTMENT OPERATIONS

One of the goals of the department manager must be the provision of optimal patient care. As stated by Vogel and associates, "A goal of every pharmacist should be to provide pharmacy services consistently according to the highest quality standards of practice currently accepted within the profession."[3] The authors also expressed the belief that quality assurance provides a means of increasing the acceptance of these (clinical) services as a necessary component of quality health care in hospitals." Whether distributive, managerial, or clinical activities are being considered, quality assurance provides the most effective method of meeting and ensuring consistency, competence, and effectiveness of services.

For example, improvements in department efficiency can easily be revealed using QA techniques. One of the most frequent proofs involves the reduction of department inventories. An audit will demonstrate drugs with low utilization, those that represent high inventory expenditures, and those that are prescribed inappropriately. Correction of these situations can produce substantial inventory reductions. For example, a three-year retrospective study of cephalosporin antibiotics in one university hospital led to a change from cephalothin, administered four times a day, to cefazolin, to be given three times a day.[4] A concomitant savings of $5,500 was realized (which comprised 10 percent of the injectable cephalosporin expenditures).

In another study, the act of observing performance led to improvement in technique.[5] When pharmacists and technicians were observed as they compounded intravenous admixtures, accuracy and aseptic controls improved. The researchers concluded that quality assurance is needed to ensure consistent quality of intravenous admixtures.

Another aspect of routine operations, that of record keeping, also requires periodic review. Are required records retrievable? Why wait until the drug enforcement officer asks to see records for purchasing and dispensing of controlled substances to obtain the answer to that question? Pharmacy records are legal evidence. QA standards should facilitate maintenance, storage, retrieval, and destruction of required records. Finally, in the event that they are required for legal purposes, records must be made legible, not only when in use, but also during the period of storage.[6]

BENEFITS OF QUALITY ASSURANCE TO THE HOSPITAL

Many of the aforementioned results can be used to "sell" the concept of quality assurance to those who have to conduct the assessments. There are, however, other documented advantages that may be realized when a QA program is implemented.

Consolidation of monitoring functions has resulted in reduced duplication of effort and decreased frequency of committee meetings, thus saving both time and staff resources.[7] The QA program can become "the hub of the wheel around which all quality-related activities revolve, and from which techniques for evaluating and improving care evolve."[8]

QA programs enable professionals to become interested in identifying and solving problems for improved patient care. Practitioners and managers are motivated to use their creativity in adapting available resources answering new needs. Therefore, quality assurance can be a cost-effective methodology.

This awareness of cost containment leads to another documented achievement: the cost of implementing some comprehensive QA programs proved to be *less* than the cost of maintaining previous evaluation activities.[9] Shanahan reported that two hospitals were able to maintain the cost of QA activities over a five-year period, at 1 percent of the total operating budget of the facilities!

When 15 hospitals in west central Ohio participated in area-wide medical care evaluation studies, they identified four general benefits of their monitoring system:[10]

1. Criteria were developed by a larger group of medical experts than is usually available in one hospital.
2. A neutral and objective review of services was possible.
3. Specialty practice areas could be emphasized in a manner appropriate for both small and large hospitals.
4. Topic-based studies of ancillary services were developed, which facilitated comparisons of physicians' practice patterns.

Reeder also pointed out that the area-wide studies fostered discovery and reporting of problems that had previously been ignored. The objectivity of the review committee was another advantage, since physicians from each hospital were represented.[11]

When practitioners participate in the QA activities (e.g., the drawing up of their own monitoring criteria) knowledge of the subject under study increases.[12] The professionals must consult the literature, seek expert opinions, and refer to their own clinical experiences, thus adding to the available body of knowledge.

Markus cautions that methods used to ensure the quality of care must also ensure the professional freedom of the practitioner as well. Evaluation studies should allow the integration of knowledge about diseases, the definition of important aspects of appropriate care, the encouragement of good record keeping, the requirement that practitioners look at their actions systematically, and the recognition of the difference between what they are actually doing and what they think they are doing.[13] Markus concludes, "Ultimately, QA activities should be regarded as primarily educational, a means whereby practitioners can strive to improve their own skills in the interest of improved patient care."[14] Achievement of the results listed above will provide the hospital with documented improvements in services. The hospital can use the resulting evidence to build and sustain a good reputation in the community. The enhanced reputation leads to a higher level of personnel seeking employment, resulting in better services to the patient.[15] Once more, quality assurance facilitates a cycle of events, ending in safer, more effective health care services.

BENEFITS OF QUALITY ASSURANCE TO THE PATIENT

Restoration of a patient's health is the goal of hospitalization. Those providing care are obligated to create a safe environment for the patient. Furthermore, the employees of an institution also deserve a wholesome working atmosphere. The entire concept of risk management evolved as a method for reducing liability, resulting from the presence of inappropriate facilities and services. Implementation of QA programs that include risk management functions has demonstrated reduced frequency of compensable incidents and reduced liability insurance premiums.[16]

Another positive result of QA activities was described by Skillicorn.[17] The usual length of hospital stay for patients waiting to be discharged from one hospital to nursing homes was 40 days. Investigation of the situation showed that there was a lack of cooperation among the services that handled this group of patients. A systematic approach was developed to handle dismissals. In two years, the length of stay was reduced more than 50 percent to 19 days. Furthermore, 70 percent of the patients went to their own homes rather than to nursing homes. The interest in the patients' welfare, sparked by the review of services, led to better care planning while the patient was hospitalized. The ultimate outcome was a dramatic improvement in both the services being provided and the attitude of the providers. Positive psychological and emotional effects were also achieved by the patients involved in the experiment.

The fact that good patient care can reduce the length of hospital stay was also discussed by Stewart.[18] He commented that criteria based on the illness of the patients and the intensity of the services provided could reduce the length of a patient's stay in a community hospital as much as 15 percent.

Another vivid example of a significant contribution to health care took place in England and Wales. A British study on maternal mortality led to the development of outcome criteria for obstetrical care. A drop in maternal mortality resulted.[19]

When audits of ancillary services are conducted, they may produce decreased hospital bills for patients by reducing the number of diagnostic tests, cost of drugs, and length of stay.[20] Consumers are becoming more aware of their rights as patients. The federal government has begun to explore competition among health care providers and insurers as a means to reduce costs. Competition may also become a method for stimulating continued improvements in service levels. If practitioners and health care institutions were required to release technical information about patient care to the public, then consumers would exert pressure on the providers to improve performance.[21] It has also been proposed that linking the quality of care to the rate of reimbursement for services would have a substantial impact on upgrading the execution of health care activities.

CHANGES IN ATTITUDE

Still another demonstrable advantage of QA programs is the improvement in the attitude of those providing patient care. Proving that one is performing well is a major accomplishment för any employee. Having one's superiors receive proof of the quality further encourages the employee to expend the required effort.

Improvement in physician performance was the end product of the area-wide study reported by Reeder, as described previously. However, results of these performance appraisals also served as an incentive for change by the medical practitioners.[22]

The subject of attitude was addressed by Skillicorn, who said that quality should be defined in terms of the attitude that perfection can be achieved; an error in direct patient care is not acceptable.[23] The transition in attitudes toward medical care evaluation among the medical staff at San Jose Hospital led to the performance of audits "not just because they are required." Since actual patient care has been evaluated, the QA team has even been requested to conduct audits![24]

Much has been said throughout this book about "patient care." By placing the emphasis on *caring*, professionals can truly demonstrate an interest in the welfare of the patient. A genuine concern for solving problems, coupled with willingness to implement corrective actions, are ways in which a hospital employee can exhibit the principles of high quality patient care.

THE FUTURE OF QUALITY ASSURANCE

Past history has clearly demonstrated that health care institutions were not providing the level of service that the consumer had a right to expect. A situation such as the nationwide recall of contaminated intravenous solutions, which took place in 1971, cannot be permitted to recur.[25] Clearly, this incident and other similar occurrences demonstrate the need for quality assurance.

The 1980s ushered in the beginning of national recognition of quality assurance as the JCAH began enforcing the new standards focused on this area of health care. At a symposium on quality assurance held at the Commission headquarters in Chicago in February 1981, the "coming of age" of quality assurance was discussed.[26] At that meeting the opinion was expressed that during the 1970s it became rational and appropriate to embrace the JCAH standards on quality assurance. It was also stated that continued support of the health care professions should lead to the continued evolution of quality assurance in the 1980s.

There are many internal and external factors that affect the direction that health care might take in the future. By analyzing current trends and extrapolating them logically it is possible to suggest future trends for quality assurance. One of the most dramatic changes that can be expected will be stimulated by computerization in virtually every health discipline. As routine tasks are assumed by the computer, more time will be spent in clinical activities. More importantly, the computer can offer technical support for clinical functions, such as patient monitoring, drug interaction screening, and kinetic dosing. A vast, new area of computerized quality assurance will be needed to prevent access to confidential data by unauthorized individuals. Techniques will also be required to guarantee access to active or inactive data, for use as legal evidence, or as a source for audit procedures.

A grass-roots movement among pharmacists, away from strictly distributive activities and toward the clinical arena, has already begun. In order to reallocate staffing to participate clinically, the manager must be able to document that all other functions are operating optimally. Quality assurance provides the required proof to justify this transition.

Another trend in hospitals is the development of group activities such as purchasing councils and area-wide performance evaluation. As health care institutions learn to disregard their differences and pool their resources, large bodies of knowledge can be developed that could be accessible to all participants. On a smaller scale this same effect takes place within the confines of a single institution—when QA committees coordinate all monitoring activities and reduce duplication of effort. Economic conditions have forced professionals to work together. The by-product of their efforts is a unity of purpose: the identification and solution of problems that have been impeding the achievement of optimal patient care.

As government programs reduce financial allocations for health related services, providers must find increasingly creative methods of attracting funding sources. If a reimbursement agent such as an insurance company has to select the services for which it will pay, it follows that the services that have documented quality will be looked on more favorably. As competition increases among providers for the consumer's health care dollar, the professional who can demonstrate efficacy and safety will have the edge over other professionals.

Another spin-off of decreased federal spending is the extinguishing of the Professional Standards Review Organizations (PSROs) that fulfilled the "watch dog" role in health care in the 1970s. Because the JCAH accredits hospitals for three years, a long period can elapse before anyone conducts a review of compliance to standards in the institution. An ongoing problem-focused QA program, however, will fill the resulting void. Medicare is also lengthening the intervals between hospital inspections. Quality assurance, on the other hand, although not yet required by Medicare, provides similar benefits in any hospital, regardless of its size, location, ownership, or accrediting organization.

It seems apparent that quality assurance is here to stay as the foundation for growth and development of health care in the future.

NOTES

1. "Symposia Supports Philosophy of QA Standard," *Perspectives,* May/June 1981, pp. 9-10.
2. Robert L. Kaufman et al., "Medication Discharge Counseling Program Developed by Pharmacists," *Hospitals* 52 (1978): 89-92.
3. David P. Vogel et al., "The Quality Assurance of Professional Staff," *Current Concepts in Hospital Pharmacy Management,* Summer 1981, pp. 8-17.
4. M.W. Noel and J. Paxinos, "Cephalosporins: Use Review and Cost Analysis," *American Journal of Hospital Pharmacy* 35 (1978): 933-935.
5. Lonnie H. Sanders et al., "Evaluation of Compounding Accuracy and Aseptic Techniques for IV Admixtures, *American Journal of Hospital Pharmacy* 35 (1978): 531-536.
6. Neil Davis, "Permanent Readable Records," editorial, *Hospital Pharmacy* 17, no. 2 (1982): 59.
7. "Symposia Supports Philosophy of QA Standard," pp. 9-10.
8. Maryanne Shanahan, "Patient Care Evaluation: Coming of Age in the 80s," *Quality Review Bulletin* 7, no. 4 (1981): 10-11.
9. Ibid.
10. Margaret Page Reeder, "The Benefits of Area-wide Quality Review," letter, *Quality Review Bulletin,* December 1981, pp. 2-3.
11. Ibid.
12. A.C. Markus, "Quality Assurance—Panacea or Trojan Horse?" *Quality Review Bulletin,* February 1981, pp. 21-22.
13. Ibid.
14. Ibid.
15. Cecelia K. Golightly, *Creative Problem Solving for Health Care Professionals* (Rockville, Md.: Aspen Systems Corp., 1981), p. 122.
16. Bernard L. Brown, Jr., *Risk Management for Hospitals—A Practical Approach* (Rockville, Md.: Aspen Systems Corp., 1979), p. 114.
17. Stanley A. Skillicorn, *Quality and Accountability* (San Francisco: Editorial Consultants, Inc., 1980), p. 25.

18. Jesse H. Stewart, "The Effect of Quality Assurance Efforts on Patient Care," *Topics in Hospital Pharmacy Management* 1, no. 3 (1981): 11-19.

19. Markus, "Quality Assurance—Panacea or Trojan Horse," pp. 21-22.

20. Reeder, "The Benefits of Area-wide Quality Review," pp. 2-3.

21. Barbara Wendorf, ed., "Is Quality Assurance Really Worth It?" *Quality Review Bulletin* 7, no. 2 (1981): 23-28.

22. Reeder, "The Benefits of Area-wide Quality Review," pp. 2-3.

23. Skillicorn, *Quality and Accountability*, p. 25.

24. Ibid., p. 24.

25. W.M. Heller, "On Maturing," *American Journal of Hospital Pharmacy* 29 (1972): 50.

26. "Symposia Supports Philosophy of QA Standard, May/June 1981, pp. 9-10.

Index

B

C

D

E

N

O

About the Authors

MARLENE LAMNIN has been the Director of Quality Assurance for HPI Hospital Pharmacies, Inc., since 1979. Her responsibilities include administration of the QA program for all of the hospital pharmacies, intravenous therapy teams, materiel management departments, and home health care facilities managed by HPI. She has spoken on the topic of quality assurance at many local, state, and national seminars for health care professionals. Also included in the scope of her professional activities is the production of audiovisual in-service programs used in the HPI contract facilities. Mrs. Lamnin received her bachelor's degree in pharmacy from the Philadelphia College of Pharmacy and Sciences. Her experiences in hospital pharmacy range from staff duties to administrative functions, including the establishment of intravenous admixture and surgery satellite pharmacy services. She has published articles in *Southern Hospitals, American Journal of Hospital Pharmacy,* and *Topics in Hospital Pharmacy Management.* She is licensed to practice pharmacy in California, Texas, and Pennsylvania. She holds memberships in the American, Texas, and California Societies of Hospital Pharmacists, National Association of Quality Assurance Professionals, and the Patient Care Assessment Council.

GARY L. SNODGRASS is Director of Clinical Services for HPI Hospital Pharmacies, Inc. His primary responsibilities include expansion of clinical services and the development and implementation of a certification process for clinical programs and practitioner competency. Dr. Snodgrass formerly held the position of Director of the Clinical Pharmacy Program, University of Rhode Island. He has served on the faculties of the University of Rhode Island, Brown Medical School, and the University of Illinois. Dr. Snodgrass received his bachelor's degree in pharmacy from the University of Nebraska. He worked two years on his master's degree in medicinal chemistry at the same university and received his doctorate from the University of Cincinnati. He completed his residency in pediatric clinical pharmacy at Children's Hospital Medical Center, Cincinnati. While on the faculty of the University of Illinois, he received a master's degree in medical education and completed a fellowship at the Center for Educational Development, Chicago.